Bioethics

Bioethics

Catastrophic Events in a Time of Terror

Howard B. Radest

LEXINGTON BOOKS

A division of
ROWMAN & LITTLEFIELD PUBLISHERS, INC.
Lanham • Boulder • New York • Toronto • Plymouth, UK

LEXINGTON BOOKS

A division of Rowman & Littlefield Publishers, Inc.
A wholly owned subsidiary of The Rowman & Littlefield Publishing Group, Inc.
4501 Forbes Boulevard, Suite 200
Lanham, MD 20706

Estover Road
Plymouth PL6 7PY
United Kingdom

British Library Cataloguing in Publication Information Available

Library of Congress Cataloging-in-Publication Data

Radest, Howard B.
Bioethics: catastrophic events in a time of terror / Howard B. Radest.
p. cm.
Includes bibliographical references and index.
ISBN 978-0-7391-3527-3 (cloth: alk. paper)
ISBN 978-0-7391-3529-7 (e-book)
1. Disaster medicine—Moral and ethical aspects. 2. Medical ethics. 3. Bioethics. I. Title.
RA645.5.R33 2009
174'.957—dc22 2009004316

Printed in the United States of America

∞™ The paper used in this publication meets the minimum requirements of American National Standard for Information Sciences—Permanence of Paper for Printed Library Materials, ANSI/NISO Z39.48-1992.

For our grandchildren,
Brendan, Colin, Emma, Kara, Jes, and Luca.
May they grow up to live in a time of peace!

Contents

Preface

In a lifetime, we will surely experience crisis, disaster, and catastrophe, natural and man-made. The former, like tsunami or the movement of tectonic plates, lacking intentionality, are just happenings. But catastrophe teaches us that all too often we are nature's partners. Where and how we build our homes, for example, converts flood and earthquake into catastrophe. How we invest our resources minimizes or increases their effects. The adequacy or inadequacy of our preparation and skill turns nature's events into human disasters. Our choices and our behavior play their roles. We are, thus, not simply victims, although it is sometimes a comfort to think of ourselves that way. Unavoidably, therefore, we face problems of moral agency and also questions of responsibility. With us, right and wrong and good and evil enter the scene.

Complicating the picture is the time in which we live. We have capabilities that enable us to respond more and more effectively to nature's events. We erect buildings, as Tokyo demonstrates, that are proof against all but the most violent earthquakes. We construct levees and dams, as the Dutch have taught us, that, quite literally, hold back the seas. We have cures that defeat epidemic or at least minimize its effects and decrease its casualties. At the same time, we—particularly, we Americans—seem to enjoy the illusion of omnipotence. For every problem, we *know* there is a solution. We think to impose our will on the world, to make it our possession, our object and our instrument. Hubris and power are twin features of modernity.

Complicating the picture even more—although it is not clear how long-lived it will be—is what I call a "time of terrorism." We add new and inventive forms of catastrophe. Hiroshima and Nagasaki are its reality and its symbol. Global terrorism is only its most recent expression. But, as we shall see, terrorism is not encapsulated in the event, the bomb exploding on train or bus, the plane destroying a building. Terrorism is also a matter of consciousness. Dread exaggerates terror's dimensions. Real enough in the blood that it sheds, the deaths that it inflicts, and the destruction that it causes, terrorism is also a distraction. For some, it is but another methodology of power. Counterterrorism and terrorism are partners, too.

It is with these thoughts in mind that I set out to prepare this essay. It is a modest effort focusing on some, but only some, of the features of this contemporary environment. Yet, I trust that my project will be illustrative and, in its own right, a useful attempt to deal with the role of bioethics amid the realities of the catastrophic in a time of terrorism.

About three years ago, Harvey Kayman, MD, a friend and at the time fellow member of the Ethics Committee of the South Carolina Medical Association, pointed out that preparations for catastrophic events and, in particular, for terrorist disasters, did not address the moral issues that were bound to arise. Quarantine, for example, would pose problems of civil liberties. Triage would pose problems of equity and equality. Treatment would pose problems of autonomy, confidentiality, and informed consent. National security would pose problems of communication and transparency. Authority would pose problems of democratic participation and accountability. To be sure, clinical and public health practices are sensitive to these problems. Yet, in reviewing documents like "Emergency Preparedness Core Competencies," I find that ethical competency is not among them.[1] Granting the tempo imposed on us by emergency, this neglect is understandable. Yet, on reflection, it seemed to us that ethical preparedness also has a role to play. For Dr. Kayman and me, this became even more urgent in a time of terrorism. Ethics in short is not a luxury.

As we talked, other questions began to shadow the conversation. Would the ethical resources that are brought to "normal" clinical and public health deliberations serve under the extreme conditions likely to occur in an environment of threat and defense? We were struck by the ways in which 9/11 and a terrorist environment like a "war on terror" were shaping the way we looked at the moral situation. For better or worse, mood and consciousness were changing in the professional and in the wider communities. So, we face three related problems—the lack of attention to bioethics in public health preparedness, the differences and similarities between dealing with "normal" disaster and in dealing with disaster in a terrorist environment, and what might be done to respond to these first two problems.

We agreed that others should be brought into the conversation and that as a first step, a course of study should be developed that addressed the concerns we had identified. An interdisciplinary planning committee was brought together to explore the project.[2] For about six months, the group met regularly. The upshot was Ethics and Public Health in an Age of Terrorism, offered initially as a pilot course at the Arnold School of Public Health of the University of South Carolina in the spring of 2005. Dr. Kayman agreed to act as faculty coordinator. I was charged with organizing the curriculum. A volunteer faculty drawn primarily from the membership of the planning committee taught the twelve modules we developed. A formal evaluation reported excellent student learning outcomes. With the leadership of the Center for Public Health Preparedness, information about the course and the concerns that led to it was shared with other centers around the country and with other schools and public health agencies.

At that point, I was asked to develop a textbook for the curriculum based on our experience with the pilot program. Completed in 2006, it became available as a CD from the Center for Public Health Preparedness at the University of South Carolina. An online version of the course is available at no cost through the Center for Public Health Preparedness, State University of New York, Albany, at www.ualbanycphp.org/learning.

As the pedagogical project continued, my own reflections on the subject evolved beyond the limits of classroom and textbook. So, when Lexington Press (Rowman & Littlefield) asked if I was interested in developing a book on bioethics in a time of terrorism, I accepted the assignment willingly, although with no little hesitation about my ability to do the job. As I saw it, a philosophic description of the bioethics problem would be helpful. Intended to be read independently, it could also complement the study of the issues we had identified in the public health preparedness curriculum.

Of course, I drew on my own research for the earlier project and on the many conversations that led to it. At the same time, I explored other and related issues that transcended its parameters. I began to think of bioethics in more inclusive and expansive ways. Trained as a philosopher, I was taught that ethics was the generic discipline and that medical ethics was one of its children. But, things are changing. Medical ethics, with its clinical focus, gives way to biomedical ethics and then to bioethics. The boundaries I was used to, so neat, became less and less useful. For example, in commenting on the United Nations Educational, Scientific, and Cultural Organization's (UNESCO) 2005 declaration on bioethics, Henk ten Have wrote,

> The *Declaration on Bioethics* thus opens perspectives for action that reach further than just medical ethics and reiterates the need to place bioethics within the

> context of reflection open to the political and social world. Today, bioethics goes far beyond the code of ethics of the various professional practices concerned. It implicates reflection on the evolution of society, indeed world stability, induced by scientific and technological developments. The *Declaration on Bioethics* paves the way for a new agenda of bioethics at the international level.[3]

In pursuing my theme, I could not help but attend, among other matters, to politics, to race and culture, and to issues of human rights. Focused on the American problem, I found myself reflecting on the transnational and communal context within which American concerns had to be placed.

Naturally, in a brief essay, I needed to work within manageable limits that would at the same time do justice to the larger subject. So, I decided to focus on a few salient examples of the catastrophic, each of which illustrated the bioethics issues I wanted to write about. In searching for these I realized that there were very few examples of terrorism that would do the job. For all their differences, terrorist events are repetitious—variations on a theme of rapid and dramatic destruction. As I will report, there are very few instances of what is called bioterror and agroterror and none thus far of nuclear terror and the much fabled suitcase bomb. There is very little that is original in the terrorist repertoire. In fact, ordinariness seems almost deliberate, and inventiveness is pretty much confined to tactics. Even 9/11, for all of its trauma, with its takeover of passenger airplanes and collapsing skyscrapers, echoed in no small measure an earlier period when hijacking was the method of choice. As a result, I turned to natural events like hurricane, flood, epidemic, and pandemic. My assumption was that extreme instances of these, like Katrina or pandemic flu, would as it were come close in experience to what equivalent terrorist events might look like.

Consequently, I concluded for a book in three sections:

1. Bioethics is unable to exist comfortably within the walls of the clinic or the laboratory. The world enters both of these all uninvited. Along the way, religious, psychological, political, legal, economic, sociological, and cultural questions appear. Ethics generally, and bioethics in particular, are in the middle of this complication of processes. In this first part of the book (chapters 1, 2, and 3), then, I try to establish the context for bioethics under the modern condition.
2. Terror, if not terrorism, finds its victims, survivors, and caregivers, its heroes, villains, and fools. Yet, in a time of terrorism, nature's havoc and human villainy and error take on added import. In this second part of the book (chapters 4, 5, 6, 7, and 8), an empirical section that uses Katrina, SARS, pandemic, and anthrax to ground the discussion, I will be looking for what persists and what changes when terror becomes terrorism.

3. Terrorism is real. Yet, bioterrorism does not offer many examples and the ones it does are meager fare when compared to 9/11 or the Madrid bombings. Does this mean that bioterrorism is only an invention of politics or panic? Or does it mean that bioterrorism is an inevitability awaiting the skill of its agents? In a concluding section (chapters 9 and 10), I try to sum up what I have found and to look forward to what might happen.

A book is a social product even if it carries the name of a single author, and this one is no exception. I am neither a biologist nor a physician. So I looked to many colleagues and friends for criticism and correction and, no doubt, I will inadvertently miss acknowledging some of them. For such neglect, I ask forgiveness. Leon Bullard, MD, a scholar and practicing physician, reassured me of the adequacy of my references to biology, medicine, and public health. He reviewed each chapter and shared his comments and criticisms with me. His wife, Cheryl Bullard, is Chief Counsel for Health Services at South Carolina's Department of Health and Environmental Control. Her guidance about public health law and the legal ins and outs of emergency powers was invaluable. Gordon Haist, my philosopher colleague at the University of South Carolina, Beaufort, read the book in its penultimate form with an eye to its philosophic ideas and the coherence of my use of them. In addition, I presented selected sections to Charley Kay, professor of Philosophy, and his students in two medical ethics classes at Wofford College and learned much from our discussions. Fellow members of the South Carolina Medical Association's Ethics Committee read and discussed the materials on Dr. Pou and Katrina and reviewed my overall approach to bioethics. I was also guided by informal discussions of a number of the issues that I was dealing with that appeared on the "listserve" of the Medical School of Wisconsin. Two of its members, Maurice Bernstein, Associate Professor of Clinical Medicine at the Keck School of Medicine, University of Southern California, and Erich Loewy, Professor of Medicine at the University of California, Davis, graciously permitted me to cite them in my chapter on the Pou case. As is the custom, and surely more than a mere courtesy, I am ultimately responsible for the ideas and errors that appear in the book.

Finally, my companion and critic of some fifty-seven years, my wife, Rita, read each chapter, shared her comments and criticisms, and most importantly made my work possible by her support and encouragement. Once again, a word of gratitude is but an inadequate token of my appreciation and gratitude.

Given my subject, it may seem strange that I have dedicated this book to my grandchildren—Brendan, Colin, Emma, Kara, Jes, and Luca. But they are the future, and the dedication to them is the message I would offer as a personal conclusion. I emerge from this project with a sense of hopefulness. Difficult and painful as it is, our time of terrorism will pass as other such times have passed. And we will go on!

NOTES

1. Columbia School of Nursing, Center for Health Policy, November 2002.
2. The committee included colleagues from the USC Center for Public Health Preparedness, the Arnold School of Public Health, and the School of Law at the University of South Carolina, the Medical University of South Carolina, Clemson University, the South Carolina Department of Health and Environmental Control, the Ethics Committee of the South Carolina Medical Association, the South Carolina Area Health Education Consortium, the South Carolina House of Representatives, and two graduate students at the Arnold School of Public Health.
3. "The Activities of UNESCO in the Area of Ethics," Henk ten Have, *Kennedy Institute of Ethics Journal*, Vol. 16, No. 4, 2006, p. 341.

1

The Many Faces of Terror

AGENDA: A FIRST LOOK

We live in a time of terrorism. We face moral and political choices that are both similar to and different from those we've ordinarily had to make when catastrophes occurred. Moral ambiguity is the result. So, we need to look anew at what happens to caregivers and victims, public health and police, government and the community at large. Exploring the role of bioethics in this shifting territory is the theme of this essay. But, I do not want to overstate the problem of today's difference. That temptation is itself part of the difference.

Before there is terrorism, there is terror. Always, human beings have faced natural disasters like flood and earthquake. Pandemic too is a lesson of history. Life, we are taught over and over again—and not merely in the terrorist event—is risky and dangerous. Yet, like those who settle on the slopes of a volcano, this seems only a momentary lesson. We return to our daily round as if nothing untoward has happened, as if nothing untoward will happen. For example,

> As the United States nears the fifth anniversary of the September 11 terrorist attacks, Americans are looking back at how their lives have changed. . . . How have their spiritual lives been affected? A new study by *The Barna Group* examined data from nine national surveys, involving interviews with more than 8,600 adults, conducted right before the attacks and at regular intervals since then. The study shows that despite an intense surge in religious activity and expression in the weeks immediately following 9/11 the faith of Americans is virtually indistinguishable today compared to pre-attack conditions. Barna's tracking surveys looked at 19 dimensions of spirituality and beliefs. Remarkably, none of those

> 19 indicators are statistically different from the summer before the attacks! If the impact of 9/11 has been nearly indistinguishable in matters of faith, the event has affected Americans' psyche in other areas. Nearly two-thirds of Americans (63 percent) described themselves as "concerned about terrorist attacks."[1]

But, we do adapt, and crisis speeds the changes. Consider how we have come to live with airport screening, with public intrusion into private spaces, with a politics that reflects angst and anguish and not a little opportunism. Our emotions and attitudes clearly are affected. Like our ancestors, we formalize and ritualize our memories of catastrophe. Flood stories, for example, are found in the mythologies of many peoples. Death and suffering are persistent themes of faith and art. And 9/11's myth is being formed even as we read the names of the casualties at its anniversary. There is some corner of our consciousness that exhibits itself in the ways we are shaped by these ultimate moments. We turn to expressive performance, whose rhythm reveals that we both want to remember and resist memory. Again, 9/11 is instructive. Seven years after the event, the site of the World Trade Center still awaits its monument. At the same time,

> Since shortly after the terrorist attacks that destroyed the World Trade Center, New Yorkers have been creating impromptu shrines, memorializing the victims. People have placed photographs of the dead and missing, together with flowers and American flags, in many places, including the walls in Grand Central Terminal, Pennsylvania Station and the 42nd Street subway stop, some of the city's most heavily traveled junctions. . . . In the opinion of Stephen P. Huyler, these shrines mean that small portions of ordinary public space have become set apart, and sanctified, by what people have placed there. Such "sacred spaces," he said, "bring healing, allowing us to bridge our grief or find a form of solace, to be quiet at a time of turmoil." . . . Making shrines, he said, "is something that's natural—it comes from deep within. It's an archetypal need of mankind to create sacred space at times of great need."[2]

Catastrophe happens, and catastrophe terrorizes. To be sure, traditions assign purpose and reason to such happenings: the angry god, the malevolent demon, or the faithless community. But in a demythologized age like our own, catastrophe is also demythologized, naturalized as it were. Save Bible literalists, it has causes but not reasons. We try to temper its effects; but we expect neither to find nor to propitiate the gods who made it happen. We are, ironically, the most capable of peoples and that very capability tells us we are helpless.

Terrorism reintroduces us to a more primitive impulse, stirs a more primitive memory. With it, catastrophe, like the stories of old, regains its reasons. We have an enemy. The sorrow and regret of the natural event where we can but cope is replaced by the passions of attack and defend. Not for nothing does the metaphor "a war on terror" seize us even as we know it is false, even as we know that it is like no "war" for which history has prepared us.[3] Gone are the boundaries of tradition, the rules of battle, and, in our more "enlightened" age, the efforts to tame warfare with international covenants. Less mundane, even apocalyptic, reality is once again peopled with villains and heroes whose being and purpose are larger than the mere give and get of ordinary living. Events regain their purpose too in a chaos of falling towers and unwitting casualties. Such a mix of memory and impulse, story and facticity invites moral confusion. In a time of terrorism, mythic and symbolic motive and language become moral barriers. The "other" becomes satanic and, by inference, we are sanctified. Ethics in such an environment must struggle against the biblical impulse in order to recover the sensibilities of law and philosophy.

But that is not easy. A reviewer of the photographs of 9/11 reminds us,

> We saw photographs that week of buildings burning, stunned onlookers, dust-covered firemen. . . . The most electrifying picture I remember from that week was a snapshot by a Port Authority employee, John Labriola. . . . A handsome young fireman is ascending the stairs, his eyes open wide, perspiring, hauling gear. All week one had seen distant images of fire and smoke, but here was a shot from inside a building about to collapse, and you looked at the fireman and thought, "My God, that man is about to be crushed to death." . . . The mainstream media seized upon inspirational and patriotic images, . . . thus began a sort of mythification of the day into which George W. Bush and Rudolph Giuliani entered, bearing spears and shields. . . . "The one conclusion I came to on 9/11 is that people in the stairwell . . . really were in 'a state of grace.' They helped each other. They didn't panic," Labriola says. "Most people are basically good. I knew this, with certainty, because I had gone through the crucible."[4]

We dare not yield to the metaphysical temptation. We need to attend to the "what" and "how" of care and reconstruction. There are wounds to treat, dead to bury, land to reclaim. In catastrophe, there are moments of choice and decision. In a terrorist event, these moments multiply. Now, there are also enemies to identify, tactics and strategies to revise. Choice and decision are not, however, only technical and tactical. Practices, politics, and economics also set parameters for dealing with the event. Issues of culture and ethnicity are always present. Moral values, judgments, and decisions are unavoidable. Willingly or not, aware or not, we deal with ethical questions, often relying on moral habits that no longer suffice: what counts as good or at least as lesser evil; what counts as benefit or harm; with triage inevitable, who will benefit and who will be harmed? In the midst of chaos, we must tame the passions that blind us, finding the moral "will" to turn reaction into action.

The terror event is connected to other like events in fact and in consciousness. Prior choices and moral habits shape our responses and set the goals that determine what counts as success and failure. Of course, goals are limited if not dictated by the facts. But there are other limits. Much as technical competence is essential to effective action, so too is moral competence. Without it, "know-how" can be defeated not by technical inability but by moral failure. Thus, paying attention to the ethics of the situation is not optional. But before we can come to the matters that are at the heart of this essay, we need to establish the context in which they occur and, in particular, the way they occur for us Americans.

9/11

Sometimes, it seems that we think and act as if terrorism began on 9/11, an ironic example of American exceptionalism. Israelis, Palestinians, Iraqis, Kurds, Iranis, Arabs, British, French, Germans, Italians, Spanish, Irish, Indians, Pakistanis, Tamils, Sikhs, Sri Lankans, Liberians, Somalis, Kenyans, and Zulus—the list could go on—would tell us otherwise. We are like them but do not realize it. Even for us, although our memory is muted, terrorism has its record, as in the first attack on the World Trade Center, the near-sinking of the USS *Cole*, the deaths of more than 250 marines in Lebanon, to name but a recent few. To be sure, 9/11 has achieved iconic status among us, a symbol of virtue's vulnerability and evil's power. Politicians after 9/11 assimilate its trauma, using it to justify policy and practice—torture and "rendition," for example, or preemptive warfare—which under another condition would be unjustifiable. Preachers and pundits on the right proclaim Armageddon. On the left, they retreat to worn out excuses for the event and its perpetrators, granting them the alibis of the victim, poverty and powerlessness.

It seems as if nearly all of us are "embedded," to borrow a term of art, from the symbiotic relationship between military and media in Iraq II. This invites emotional identification with authority and power—even for those in putative opposition—with all of the control and self-censorship the term implies. Terrorism, it would seem, shapes our perceptions and our consciousness to a new obedience and a new silence. Challenge and critique, we agree in unspoken consensus, which only adds to terror's anxiety. Hence, a leadership of "either/or" seems the requirement of survival. Terrorism creates its mirror image in the terrified for whom certainty, any certainty, is preferable to a world become chaotic.

Of course, no one is untouched by 9/11, and no one is free of the destruction it forecasts. Terrorism, as it were, has already done its job, even if there is no sequel in events. We behave differently, think differently, feel differently. We may appear to return to old habits, but we have learned to live looking over our shoulder. Thus, the suspicion that attends air travel and the covert—sometimes not so covert—glances at fellow passengers of different color, tongue, and costume. Thus, too, the rhetoric of the politician on all sides and the expectations of his/her listeners.

While terrorism is elusive, terror is not. We are no strangers to it. Thor and Zeus and the Hebrew God, with their awesome presence and fearsome power, capture this dimension of the human psyche with thunder and lightening bolt. Shiva, bringing, paradoxically, wisdom and destruction, is worshipped and feared. Scripture is filled with images of terror, the hidden face of the Lord, His power revealed in the Flood, the destruction of Sodom and Gomorrah, the slaying of the Egyptian first born in Exodus. For the Christian, Revelation predicts the "end time," its coming foretold by signs and symbols promising world destruction. On a less lofty and secular plane, psychiatric couch and existential poesy are witness to terror's anxiety and its effects. All in all, catastrophe reinforces a felt arbitrariness in our experience of the world and we, creatures of memory and imagination, encounter it and tremble as we try to read its meaning.

Seizing upon terror's ubiquity, policy turns our existential condition to the advantage of terrorism and counterterrorism alike. And while these acquire new dimensions in our time—of which more later—they are surely not new. Bioterrorism has its place in history too even if the use of disease and poison as weapons is, thus far at least, rare.

> One of the first recorded incidents was in Mesopotamia, by the city-state Assyria. The Assyrians employed rye ergot, an element of the fungus *Claviceps purpurea*, which contains mycotoxins. Rye ergot was used by Assyria to poison the wells of their enemies, with limited success. Hellebore, a plant with powerful purgative and cardiac glycoside effects, was also used by the Greeks to poison the water supply during their siege of the city of Krissa.[5]

Nor is terrorism new to the American experience, although sometimes, listening to ourselves, we might think it is. Hijacked airplanes, suicide bombings, kidnappings, and assassinations are no strangers to the American story. Our history tells us we have been both victim and perpetrator of "guerilla warfare," raids on Native American communities, the seizing and killing of hostages, the destruction of peoples and not just of armies. In our own time, the U.S. State Department historian has chronicled several hundred "significant" terrorist incidents, many involving Americans, in the years between 1961 and 2003, few of them until recently on our own soil.[6] Nor are we innocent of the uses of terror, as in "scorched earth" tactics during the Civil War, the mass bombings of WWII, and "carpet bombing" in Vietnam.

Latterly, Mr. Rumsfeld, the former Secretary of Defense, as if descending from Sinai, heralded the invasion of Iraq in 2003 as "shock and awe." Becoming nature's competitor, the TV screen was filled with images of man-made lightning and sounds of man-made thunder. "Shock and awe," no doubt a phrase to capture an attentive public, was not, however, some word-spinner's invention. It referenced a strategic analysis and reflected a self-conscious decision to use its findings: terror in all its technological brilliance, as a military tactic. In their 1996 study at the National Defense University, Harlan K. Ullman and James P. Wade had identified examples of "shock and awe"—the bombing of Hiroshima and Nagasaki and blitzkrieg, to name two. Some seven years later "shock and awe" would become policy and theater all at once.

Ullman and Wade cite a striking example, even more dramatic today as a forecast of its contemporary Iraqi cousin. They write,

> Sun Tzu was brought before Ho Lu, the King of Wu, who had read all of Sun Tzu's thirteen chapters on war and proposed a test of Sun's military skills. Ho asked if the rules applied to women. When the answer was yes, the king challenged Sun Tzu to turn the royal concubines into a marching troop. The concubines merely laughed at Sun Tzu until he had the head cut off the head concubine. The ladies still could not bring themselves to take the master's orders seriously. So, Sun Tzu had the head cut off a second concubine. From that point on, so the story goes, the ladies learned to march with the precision of a drill team.
>
> The objectives of this example are to achieve Shock and Awe and hence compliance or capitulation through very selective, utterly brutal and ruthless, and rapid application of force to intimidate. Decapitation is merely one instrument. The intent here, is to impose a regime of Shock and Awe . . . directed at influencing society writ large, meaning its leadership and public, rather than targeting directly against military or strategic objectives.[7]

Terrorism thus has many faces. Nation states may resort to strategies of terror or may support quasi-independent terrorist organizations. And, lest we situate this tactic only in today's Middle East, we need to be reminded that no nation or sect is privileged to resist the temptations of terrorism. I think of the French and Indian War in the British American colonies or the Kashmir border between India and Pakistan. Nationalists—the Mau Mau in sub-Saharan Africa or the Sinn Fein in Northern Ireland—may adopt terrorism as they attempt to free themselves from colonialism and foreign occupation. Facing the overwhelming military and technical power of the modern nation-state, liberation seems to leave no other option. Left- and right-wing ideologies may lead to terrorism, too, as with the Red Brigade in twentieth-century Italy and the KKK in nineteenth-century America. Religion may proclaim "holy war" which, given the Crusades, the Irgun in British-occupied Palestine, or the Sikhs seeking autonomy in India, is not uniquely Islamist. And, of course, there are anarchic terrorists for whom chaos becomes its own reward. As instance joins instance, terrorism is both tangible in its horror and elusive in its meaning. Is "terrorist" the name of our enemies but never of us? Surely, there is moral arrogance and viciousness too hidden or not so hidden in the question and its answer.

It is not surprising that a commonly agreed upon legal definition of terrorism does not exist. Thus, the United Nations admits that

> the question of a definition of terrorism has haunted the debate among states for decades. A first attempt to arrive at an internationally acceptable definition was made under the League of Nations, but the convention drafted in 1937 never came into existence. The UN Member States still have no agreed-upon definition. Terminology consensus would, however, be necessary for a single comprehensive convention on terrorism, which some countries favour in place of the present 12 piecemeal conventions and protocols.[8]

Terrorism expert Alex Schmid suggested in a 1992 report for the then UN Crime Branch that, "if the core of war crimes—deliberate attacks on civilians, hostage taking and the killing of prisoners—is extended to peacetime, we could simply define acts of terrorism as peacetime equivalents of war crimes." Gabriel Palmer-Fernandez suggests,

> I propose, then, the following definition of the core feature of terrorism. Terrorism is the organized use of violence against civilians or their property, the political leadership of a nation, or soldiers (who are not combatants in a war) for political purposes. On this account, Robespierre, Stalin, Pol Pot, the radical environmentalists, the suicide bombers in Beirut and Saudi Arabia were terrorists. So, too, was John Brown. They killed civilians or destroyed their property or held hostages for a political purpose. We need now to determine whether what John Brown and other terrorists do is immoral.[9]

No doubt these are usable definitions. But a careful reading of these efforts to capture objectively and accurately "core features" of terrorism reveals our moral and not just our legal problems. Naming the obvious villains—Stalin, Pol Pot, et al—evokes the nod of a widely shared moral consensus and not a little self-interest. It lasts as long as we ignore the fact that terrorists can be rehabilitated when successful, as in Israel's Begin or Libya's Qaddafi. Yasir Arafat, after all, was awarded a Nobel Peace Prize. For those of us not enamored of the "war between the states," John Brown's presence in the list may come as a shock. Not of alien land and time, Palmer-Fernandez reminds us that he is a folk hero celebrated in song and fiction. "John Brown's body lies amoldering in the grave, glory, glory hallelujah, his truth is marching on!" We recognize the presence, no matter how well defended by tradition, of point of view and not of universally shared moral values.[10] It is not as easy as we so often claim to separate virtue and vice, to assign innocence and culpability, and to say what these mean "on the ground."

In *The Looming Tower: Al-Qaeda and the Road to 9/11*, Lawrence Wright makes the point in the following paragraph,

> Their motivations varied, but they had in common a belief that Islam—pure and primitive, unmitigated by modernity and uncompromised by politics—would cure the wounds that socialism or Arab nationalism had failed to heal. They were angry but powerless in their own countries. They did not see themselves as terrorists but as revolutionaries who, like all such men throughout history, had been pushed into action by the simple human need for justice. Some had experienced brutal repression; some were simply drawn to bloody chaos. From the beginning of Al Qaeda, there were reformers and there were nihilists. The dynamic between them was irreconcilable and self-destructive, but events were moving so quickly that it was almost impossible to tell the philosophers from the sociopaths. They were glued together by the charismatic personality of Osama bin Laden, which contained both strands, idealism and nihilism, in a potent mix.[11]

Finally, despite the understandable response of terror's victims, the name *terrorist* has a relativist's pedigree, an invitation to political opportunism and manipulation. Thus, yet one more moral ambiguity in the midst of the terror event.

A TIME OF TERRORISM

Terrorism in our time is marked by successive events, global and local, predictable and surprising all at once. No place is secure, no moment is safe, and no person is untouchable. Choosing up sides between vice and virtue is an ever-present temptation. Aggression is an ever-present temptation. Anger, fear, and anxiety become our companions. The ways in which we perceive, judge, decide, and act in responding to the terrorist event change. In turn, these changes reshape our moral sensitivities and our ethical judgments. It is these changes that lead me to call our moment in history a "time of terrorism." Terrorist patterns and not just localized and episodic events appear. The very geography of terrorism has altered.

Terrorism has a long and bloody history, revealed in striking fashion when we catalogue "terrorist" organizations. In the last century and the beginning of this one, there was the Ku Klux Klan in several incarnations, the Irish Republican Army, the ETA (Spain), the Front du Libération de Québec, the Palestine Liberation Organization, the Red Army Faction (Baader-Meinhof Gang, Germany), the Red Brigade (Italy), the Weathermen (U.S.), Shining Path (Peru), Hamas (Palestine), Los Macheteros (Puerto Rico), Hezbollah (Lebanon), Islamic Jihad (Egypt, Palestine), Jemaah Islamyah (Southeast Asia), Tamil Tigers (Sri Lanka) . . . and the list is incomplete.

New organizations appear and disappear. Sometimes, as with kidnappings in Iraq and Afghanistan, a terrorist "name" and claim is attached to what is plain gangsterism. In fact, it's hard to tell how many groups there are, how big or small they are, how long-lived or momentary they are. Religious and secular, nationalist and anarchic, Asian, European, Latin American, Middle Eastern, and North American, they exist. Given the uses of modern communication, they are no longer merely isolated enclaves of discontent.

Terrorist tactics takes many forms, too. Assassination, kidnapping, hostage-taking, bombing, car bombing, and hijacking name genres, not events. Always violent and indifferent to the identity of its casualties, terror's violence is as much psychological as political and military. With a few exceptions, bioterror, chemical (gas), and radiological attacks are, thus far, not a method of choice. Instead, terror's methods are ordinarily simple and direct, relying more on readily available materials, willing sacrifices like suicide bombers, and the striking and newsworthy event. Thus far at least—but there are no guarantees—nonstate tactics avoid sophisticated materials and technologies, but whether by choice or inability is unclear. Of course, it is the very ordinariness of its methods that makes terrorism accessible to just about anyone and its suppression virtually impossible. Like the dragon's teeth of myth, the capture, destruction, or disappearance of this or that terrorist cell or this or that terrorist leader is no warrant of the disappearance of terrorist activity. "Terrorists" and "terrorism" spring up just about anywhere. Their's is real or apparent grievance, real or apparent ideological conflict, real or apparent denial of justice and rights.

In part, our age requires terrorism. With the evolution of a relatively small number of major powers with mass armies and sophisticated technologies, resistance movements are unable to compete directly. Others, of course, are moved to terrorism without plan or purpose. For them, disruption of the status quo becomes a self-sustaining motivation. Terrorism becomes a type of sociopolitical theater, something its nineteenth-century ancestors, the "anarchists," would recognize. But most terrorism has its reasons as well as its motives. When it matures, it takes shape as guerilla warfare and insurgency. In response, the new *U.S. Army and Marine Field Manual* comments,

> The recent dominant performance of American military forces in major combat operations may lead many future opponents to pursue asymmetric approaches. Because America retains significant advantages in fire and surveillance, a thinking enemy is unlikely to choose to fight U.S. forces in open battle. Opponents who have attempted to do so, such as in Panama in 1989 or Iraq in 1991 and 2003, have been destroyed in conflicts that have been measured in hours or days. Conversely, opponents who have offset America's fire and surveillance advantages by operating close to civilians and news media, such as Somali clans in 1993 and Iraqi insurgents in 2005, have been more successful in achieving their aims. This does not mean that counterinsurgents do

not face open warfare. Insurgents resort to conventional military operations if conditions seem right, in addition to using milder means such as nonviolent political mobilization of people, legal political action, and strikes. Insurgency has been a common approach used by the weak to combat the strong.[12]

Historically, terrorism has been local or regional and terror events have been episodic or at least seemed to be. But with the rapid and worldwide development of inexpensive and nearly untraceable electronic technologies, global communication becomes available. Comprehensive and accessible, the new media spread the word—about events, weaponry, and techniques, about tactical successes and failures. Bigger-than-life figures, like the elusive bin Laden and organizations like Al Qaeda, become points of identity for and among the most disparate of causes and places. Ironically, we have indeed become one world.

Under modern conditions, terrorism remains pluralist. At the same time, it evolves toward a coordination of purposes, tactics, skills, and models. It becomes in ways now possible both local and international. Diverse and scattered over the globe, it is not some vast conspiracy, although there is a certain comfort in thinking that it is. Conspiracy, after all, is intelligible, even potentially manageable. Terrorism's genius, however, is precisely its lack of a center and high command and therefore its lack of vulnerability. Anyone anywhere may join in and has. And given the likelihood of resentment, a consequence of widely communicated expectations of freedom and a better life and technologies as widely available, we cannot expect terrorism to be a phenomenon of the moment.

Seen globally, terrorist events have increased in frequency and number—or is it that our knowledge of them has become more adequate and our sensitivity to them understandably heightened? For example, in the Department of State list of "Significant Terror Incidents," the decade between 1961 and 1970 identified six. Coming closer to the present, 2000 had nine, 2001 had nineteen, 2002 had forty-three, and 2003 had forty-five.[13] We live in time of terrorism and are poorly served if we become victims of a paranoid consciousness on the one hand and of blindness to global patterns on the other.

NOTES

1. "Five Years Later: 9/11 Attacks Show No Lasting Influence on Americans' Faith," *Barna Update*, Ventura, CA, 8/28/06. The Barna Group regularly reports on religious attitudes and beliefs.

2. "Shrines Serve the Need for Healing in Public Spaces," Gustav Niebuhr, *NYT*, 10/6/01.

3. War usually requires absolute clarity about identities. Who are you, and where do you stand? Friend or foe? Combatant or bystander? To whom do you owe allegiance, for whom are you willing to die, and who is responsible for your conduct? This is one reason for military uniforms: they establish collective identity in the midst of the action. Individual differences are stripped away. Allegiance is reduced to conformity.

But the battles now being fought in Lebanon represent a newer form of warfare. For Hezbollah confusion of identity is not an accident but the principal tactic: no uniforms, no separation of army and populace, no clarity about ultimate responsibility. For its opponent there are always questions. What is being hit? An apartment building or a weapons depot? A farm truck or a munitions carrier? A fighter or a civilian? And who is answerable for Hezbollah's acts?

"Labyrinthine Complexities of Fighting a Terror War," Edward Rothstein, *NYT*, 8/7/06.

4. *Watching the World Change: The Stories behind the Images of 9/11*, David Friend, Farrar, Straus, and Giroux. Reviewed by Garrison Keillor, *NYT*, 9/3/06.

5. "Bioterrorism: A Brief History," Michael B. Phillips, MD, Department of Internal Medicine, Mayo Clinic, Focus on Bioterrorism, *Northeast Florida Medicine*, 2005, p. 32.

6. *Significant Terrorist Incidents, 1961–2003: A Brief Chronology*, Historical Background, Office of the Historian, Bureau of Public Affairs, U.S. Department of State, March 2004.

7. *Project Gutenberg's Shock and Awe*, Harlan K. Ullman and James P. Wade, Command and Control Research Program (CCRP), Office of the Assistant Secretary of Defense, NDU Press Book, December 1996. Examples and comments from pp. 20–23.

8. *United Nations Crime and Drug Conventions*; Crime Commission (CCPCJ); Commission on Narcotic Drugs (CND); Global Youth Network, 2006.

9. "Terrorism, Innocence, and Justice," Gabriel Palmer-Fernandez, *Philosophy and Public Affairs*, Vol. 25, No. 3, Summer 2005, p. 24.

10. On May 21, 1856, proslavery forces from Missouri attacked the antislavery town of Lawrence, Kansas, looting stores, burning buildings, and beating residents. Three days later, John Brown, proclaiming himself the servant of the Lord, along with his group of antislavery fighters known as the Free State volunteers, sought revenge by killing five proslavery farmers along the Pottawatomie Creek. At the Doyle farm, James and his two sons were hacked to death. Mrs. Doyle, a daughter, and a fourteen-year-old son were spared. Brown and his fighters then moved on to a second farm, where Allen Wilkinson was taken prisoner, and finally to a third where William Sherman was executed. The attack on Lawrence and the subsequent killings at Pottawatomie Creek sparked a guerilla war between proslavery and antislavery forces in Missouri and Kansas that lasted several months and cost nearly two hundred lives. Fernandez, "Terrorism, Innocence, and Justice."

11. *The Looming Tower: Al-Qaeda and the Road to 9/11*, Lawrence Wright, Alfred A. Knopf, 2006, pp. 301, 304, 348–50.

12. *Counterinsurgency*, FM 3-24, June 2006. (Final Draft—Not For Implementation), pp. 1–2.

13. *Significant Terrorist Incidents*, U.S. State Department.

2

Ethics, Thick and Thin

COMMUNITY AS PATIENT

In a recent study, I concluded that clinical ethics relies on the story and the case, i.e., on the tangibility of the patient's experience and the sensitivity of the caregiver.[1] Catastrophe also lends itself to "thinking with cases." Its stories, however, are centered in communities in trouble. Its narratives are dramas of surprise, violence, suffering, heroism, cowardice, and death. We face situations we'd rather not face and must make choices we'd rather not make. Triage, in other words, is catastrophe's paradigmatic process. Each event has its own identity and stirs its own memories. At the same time, each event is a reminder and a warning. 9/11 and Katrina become symbols and not just dates and locations. They are recalled in the first-person singular—community becomes intimate—and shared, as in "I remember where I was or what I was doing when."

With narrative, the event establishes a dimension beyond the boundaries of the event itself. The story becomes a "case," a middle moment, pointing in two directions: to the experience from which it arises and to the reports by which it is classified. The latter, the cases, are deliberately impersonal. They highlight the commonalities we need for research and prediction. They reduce the story to an instance and bury it in abstraction. By contrast, a story is vivid and intense. It is "told to" and "heard by" not once but many times. Survivors and first responders make specific references to place, time, and incident. These are recognizable to the rest of us who may in turn retell the story, making it our own. Veterans, we know, tell "war stories," usually with a mixed mood of sentiment, humor, and fear. Physicians and nurses remember the special case or the difficult patient. We are all storytellers, revealing ourselves in anecdote and epic alike.

Mary Faith Marshall catches my meaning when she writes,

> Years ago, when I was writing a chapter on micro and macro allocation for the first edition of *Introduction to Clinical Ethics*, I thought long and hard about tragic choices. I wanted to open the chapter with a paradigm case; with a seemingly impossible dilemma. . . . I wanted to assert, from the get-go and in a graphic way, the nature of moral dilemmas, the fact that they don't involve, as Joseph Fletcher put it, "Sunday school ethics." To put forth Hegel's notion that tragedy is not the simplistic collision of good and evil, but involves the "headachy" business of choosing between competing goods, or competing evils . . . I wanted to ensure that those who might "do" clinical ethics . . . understood the emotional and personal liabilities for all concerned in ethics case consultation—to veer prospective consultants away from the pitfalls of hubris, complacency, and self-satisfaction.[2]

The clinical event is a transaction between individuals—the fabled doctor/patient relationship is its model. The scale is local and personal. In catastrophe, stories are magnified. Political, communal, and cultural institutions join clinical description, as in the move from medical care to public health. The "strangers at the bedside," no longer strangers, now claim a legitimate presence. Public officials, lawyers, law enforcement, clerics, reporters, etc., are essential actors along with caregivers and public health workers. With terrorism, the military and security agencies join the array. The scene is crowded, contradictory. Emergency will set limits to decision-making. Budgets will set limits to choices. Culture and practice will shape perceptions and reactions. At the same time these varied institutions will be regarded, often inappropriately, as intruders.[3]

Of course, there are exceptional events everywhere—the test case in the law, the "classic" case in the clinic, the paradigm case in public health. Their very identification tells us that something other than the particular event is involved. Naming (e.g., "Baby Fay" or "Schiavo") signals their dimensionality as more than themselves. Similarly, Katrina and 9/11 name models of catastrophe, natural and man-made. Stories, in many-layered fashion, recall what happened, bringing the event into a relived present. The epistemic scene that the story portrays precedes and forecasts how perception, memory, and thought will report and interpret. Not least of all, it invites the transition from narrative to poetry (i.e., ultimately, the emergence of recurring symbols out of dramatic events has aesthetic quality).

TERROR'S GRAMMAR

In the chapters ahead—Katrina, Dr. Pou, SARS, pandemic, etc.—we will notice many ways of characterizing terror events. We may classify them as natural,[4] or as the result of human ignorance, error, or sabotage, i.e., as in the nature of things, or as stupid, careless, or vicious. Terrorist events may be any or all of these, but above all they are intentional—they aim to achieve some end-in-view, tactical or strategic or psychological. Except for those religionists and ideologues for whom history is eschatological drama, intention is absent in natural events like flood and earthquake. Terrorist events are thus distinguishable, i.e., as religious, ideological, political, or personal. We identify them by the intent and motive of their actors, also religious, ideological, political, or personal.

The terrorist event is also distinguished by its drama, like car bombs and beheadings. These serve as messages and, given our mass media, are effective and widely circulated messages. Almost surreal, ordinary objects—bicycles, trucks, automobiles, airplanes, packages, suitcases, book matches, box cutters—are used for nonordinary ends. This inventiveness reinforces terror. A toaster or a computer becomes a weapon. A shoe turns into a bomb. Objects of daily life become untrustworthy—as we are reminded when told not to carry toothpaste or aftershave onto an airplane. Terrorist events have targets and not just victims. They are, with the exceptions of assassinations, anonymous, collective. In turn, persons become objects too, counters in someone else's intentions. The terrorist effect is enhanced. Anonymity's message is clear: I am not a person. Nothing I am or can do will prevent me from becoming terror's object. Innocence, as in "innocent bystander," is denied.

Terrorist events may be differentiated by the amount of destruction they cause and the number of casualties they inflict. They are organized or chaotic, a continuing strategy or isolated acts. Technical sophistication, e.g., biological, chemical, explosive, or radiological, is yet another way of classifying events. No doubt, too, the list can be extended and, as terrorism evolves, it will be.

Experience is intimate and "owned." Of course, given that we are social animals, ownership becomes, more often than not, shared ownership; hence, the significance of the story. To be sure, references to experience in general (e.g., the experience of terror) are useful as conceptual placeholders. If, however, we mistake this generality for reality, we get, as Alfred North Whitehead put it in another context, instances of "misplaced concreteness." In our anxiety to tame terrorism, however, to make it intelligible, we lose sight of terror's intimacy and particularity. We are driven to orderliness and thereby to forgetfulness. Generals, we say, "fight the last war all over again." Communities and their agents meet the last terrorist event all over again.

We fit the terrorist event to a pattern—an age of terrorism, a war on terror, a time of terrorism, etc. Certainly, these phrases have rhetorical uses. But, whether such patterns exist is something to be demonstrated, not assumed. As likely, they are advanced for ideological, strategic, psychological, or propaganda purposes. With the appearance of Al Qaeda and the availability of the Internet, it is easy to perceive all terrorist events everywhere as interconnected. As often as not, we agree without asking for much in the way of evidence. We may even hear the claim that the very absence of evidence demonstrates the wiliness of the conspirators. At the same time, having a named enemy with intentions, motives, and plans is strangely comforting. We can now predict the political, economic, military, and psychological consequences of conspiracy and attack. With that, we know—or think we know—what to do. We've had enemies before; we've dealt with enemies before.

To be sure, analysis, interpretation, and prediction can illuminate both natural and terrorism events. The experience of flood or pandemic helps us respond to bombing attacks or anthrax letters. The lessons we learn in dealing with terrorism in London, Mumbai, or Nairobi can be adapted to Chernobyl or Graniteville. SARS can prepare us for bioterror. Gratefully, we are convinced that terrorism is not alien ground.

As we describe a terrorist event, we reveal our own intentions and motives, some transparent, others hidden, and still others self-deluding. We facilitate analysis, interpretation, and preparation, but we also invite error and confusion. By focusing on scale, a nuclear attack for example, we are able to calculate the resources we will need and the likelihood that they will be available. We may conclude that the best that can be done is evacuation or, depending on the size of things, that the priority is protection of "first responders" in order to deal with inevitable casualties afterward. The story of SARS or of the recent failed effort to inoculate first responders against smallpox introduces us to bioterror at a moment when the actual event hardly exists.[5]

Technical and scientific procedures tend to be explicit and structured, e.g., as in the clinical "standard of care" or the military "standard operating procedure." Ethical considerations are less accessible. Indeed, doing ethics in the midst of disaster will probably be seen as "unrealistic." Yet, the "realist" pose ignores the fact that technical judgments are not self-evident but reflect cultural and moral values. A religious community may choose its priorities differently from a secular community. Sacred spaces may be protected even at the cost of added casualties. Democratic and authoritarian societies will have different moral priorities. Deciding who shall live and who shall die will rely on different social values.

Choices emerge from existing perceptions and shape future ones. Identifying a terrorist event as a military act produces one kind of response. Identifying it as a crime produces another and different response. The Guantanamo confusion over the status of its prisoners exhibits this difference. A "war on terrorism" invites the notion of "prisoners of war." So, we debate the relevance of the rules of war, the Geneva Conventions, and the Uniform Code of Military Justice to "nonstate" belligerents. Naming an event "criminal," on the other hand, calls for due process, the rules of evidence, trial by jury, the right to face one's accusers, etc. A given choice will involve the actual or implicit rejection of other possibilities. For example, classification as a "nonstate" combatant with the implication that the terrorist is literally an "outlaw" excludes treatment ordinarily accorded to "citizens." Both military and criminal characterizations undervalue or even violate public health or clinical norms (e.g., the resort to "extreme interrogation," indefinite incarceration, the priority given to attack and defense rather than to treatment).

Characterizations are imperfect, and so choices are imperfect. The "same" event will have multiple meanings and call for multiple responses. Characterizations are also backward looking—we have encountered similar events in the past or think we have. But we *will* be surprised. For example, caregivers and hospitals mobilized for catastrophe in order to treat 9/11's wounded only to find that there were massive fatalities and relatively few wounded. We needed morgues not clinics, pathologists not clinicians. Making moral sense becomes, on this account, difficult and frustrating. It is a skeptic's project.

Characterizations are finally instrumental. There is no master description that can finally capture the terrorism event. Nor can any particular description be normative for others "like" it without risking distortion in our understanding and ineffectiveness in our response. *Terrorism*, the word itself, is a situated characterization with its limitations and ambiguities. Ignorance or error will sometimes look like sabotage. Biological attack may look like pandemic, and pandemic may look like biological attack.

Even so seemingly self-evident a distinction as that between the natural and the man-made has its ambiguities. We human beings are not infrequently nature's unwitting if minor allies. Thus, we build cities on coastal plains and fault lines, dam up rivers, and invite the wind's destruction by clearing natural windbreaks. For example,

> Rising ocean temperatures linked by some studies to tropical storms are very likely a result of global warming caused by greenhouse gas emissions. . . . [R]esearchers compared a century of observed temperature changes with those produced in more than eighty computer simulations of how oceans respond to natural and human influences on the climate. . . . [They] said [that] the only warming influence that could explain the changes in the oceans was the

> buildup of heat-trapping smokestack and tailpipe gases in the air. . . . "Even under modest scenarios for emissions, we're talking about sea surface temperature changes in these regions of a couple of degrees," . . . [Benjamin D. Santer, lead author of the study] said. "That's much larger than anything we've already experienced, and that is worrying."[6]

A flood will have its man-made features too, as we'll see in our discussion of Katrina. Responses to the Southeast Asia tsunami were shaped by a community caught up in terrorism and counterterrorism.

> Although this catastrophe was unusually vast, it was a classic natural disaster in several ways. First, it is not yet complicated by war or terrorism. Indeed, both civil conflicts that were under way in the affected region, in northern Sri Lanka and in Aceh, Indonesia, have quieted in the midst of this mass distress. The situation in Aceh, however, appears to be fluid. Early reports that the various armed parties and government forces were working together to bring aid to the populations in need are now being overtaken by news of increasing tension. . . . In the event that government hostility to outside help begins to interfere with the relief effort, this disaster could become a complex emergency.[7]

Terrorist events tempt us to confuse what something is with what it is called. By naming, we combat our vulnerability. As our less industrialized ancestors understood, naming is power. It establishes the authority and status of the givers of the name. For both terrorism and counterterrorism, reputations and powers are at stake. Interests are in conflict. Both invite political and social manipulation. Naming adds potency to the invitation.

In the terrorism event, language may mask rather than communicate, as when we use "collateral damage" and "rendition" to blur suffering, death, and torture. Indeed, terms that hide rather than reveal are typical of threat and anxiety. To further confound us, this hiddenness may be either a mistake or a lie. After all, we have ample experience both of self-delusion and Machiavellian politics.

Yet, events do not speak for themselves. Language is unavoidable; abstraction is unavoidable. We cannot, like the nominalist philosophers in *Gulliver's Travels,* carry with us ever-larger sacks of objects so that we can evade words by pointing to them. The singularity of the event, however, does not foreclose our ability to learn from it. Borrowing both method and epistemology from the arts, events too can be identified on the basis of form, style, or subject matter. We can recognize *genre.* More intuitive than formal, genre admits the legitimacy of intuition and sensibility. We acknowledge kinships while recognizing individualities. This allows us to establish policies and practices that carry over from one event to another yet open enough to allow for the nuanced and the unexpected. With that in mind, terrorism may be best understood as a genre—the terror event, its expression.

Epistemology is thus completed by aesthetics. As Emerson, no doubt unfair to scientists if not to the sciences, put it,

> Science was false by being unpoetical. It assumed to explain a reptile or mollusk, and isolated it—which is hunting for life in graveyards. . . . The metaphysician, the poet, only sees each animal form as an inevitable step in the path of creating mind. The Indian, the hunter, the boy with his pets, have sweeter knowledge of these than the savant. . . . The poet gives us eminent experiences only—a god stepping from peak to peak, not planting his foot but on a mountain. Science does not know its debt to imagination.[8]

BIOETHICS[9]

Not for nothing is the human being called the "ethical animal." A creature of memory and imagination, we seem hardwired to understand the distinction between "is" and "ought." We recognize claims of good and evil, of right and wrong. We feel shame, make excuses, and attribute praise and blame. None of this, of course, insures that we will behave ethically, only that we can understand the moral process.

Ethical ideas and values arise in social, political, cultural, and psychological contexts. In Western societies, however, ethics is typically presented in nonhistorical form, a tradition reaching back to Plato's notion that "ideas" are found in their perfection in the "heaven beyond the heavens." To be sure, Aristotle, his student and fellow Athenian, was a moral empiricist and psychologist and challenged his teacher. But I suspect, we are still more Platonist than Aristotelian.

Influenced by this Platonism and by the legalism of Scripture as well, ethical ideas are set apart from the realities of give and get. They seem to stand apart, independent of events, needs, passions, and temperaments. For example, it is only recently that clinical ethics in considering issues like "futility" has acknowledged the moral legitimacy of considering the economics of care in making treatment decisions. Following the pragmatist's insight, a careful look tells us that ethics, however formulated, responds to actual problems of time, place, and person.

Ethics surely has its rarefied theories. Briefly summed up: *utility*, an ethics that focuses on outcomes, benefits, and costs; *duty*, an ethics that focuses on what ought to be done for its own sake; *virtue*, an ethics that focuses on character and conduct. Ethical ideas may be rooted in religious life views, as with Roman Catholic *natural law theory*. More recently, *feminism* and *ethnicity* have emerged since the 1960s as moral themes in response to social and political developments.

Some ethical ideas will lead to rules like the Ten Commandments, to *maxims* like those of Immanuel Kant's "pure practical reason," or to professional codes of conduct. Experience may generate moral guidelines like *an ethics of caring,* which are less legalistic than rules, maxims, and codes. A particularly apt approach for probing the moral dimensions of the terrorist event is *principlism.* Developed as a way of dealing with clinical ethics, it provides reliable criteria for moral judgment in crisis. Building on a "common morality" that is both its strength and its weakness, four principles are identified: autonomy, beneficence, nonmalificence, and justice.

For example, autonomy requires that we respect the personal moral decision. In the terrorist event where calculations of the "greatest good for the greatest number" make for sensible policy, autonomy cautions us against absolutizing moral calculation in the name of emergency. At the very least, we must be prepared to give morally defensible reasons for our failure, however understandable, to honor dissenting conscience and belief. Justice alerts us to a fair distribution of burdens and benefits in the burden-laden environment of the catastrophic event. In short, "principlism" is a constant reminder of human dignity and respect, i.e., the values characteristic of both caregiving professionalism and democratic community in situations where ignoring or minimizing these may be necessary.

Finally, these principles allow the moral "amateur" (e.g., physicians, nurses, social workers, first responders) to make moral sense without requiring elaborate preparation for which time and training are simply unavailable. The principles lack the rigidity of moral codes on the one side and avoid the endless probing that ethical inquiry requires on the other. They are, as their authors identify them, "middle level concepts," and in practice are better than good enough.[10] In a time of terrorism, they serve a dialectical need, creating a necessary tension between urgency and decency.

At the same time, the four principles illustrate the problem of cultural habit, i.e., they wear the costume of universality while clearly reflecting the logical neatness of Western tradition. In fact, the boundaries between moral territories change in response to events, histories, and futures. Today, ethics must take account of an inclusive definition of persons, i.e., the status of women, children, and ethnic minorities. Animal-rights theorists advocate an even more radical view of inclusion. New kinds of communities appear as we move from family and clan to an urban and technological society. We are barraged with information that we can neither absorb nor validate so, while truth telling remains a moral good in principle, it becomes an actual moral puzzle over and over again. International trade has its own moral dilemmas. When and where, for example, is a "bribe" a bribe? Travel adds new content to moral experience. The biological sciences probe areas once thought inviolable, like the nature of human nature or redefining the meanings of death.

Globalism raises issues of comparative ethics and challenges the habit of moral universalism. A recent study concluded,

> All three of our exploratory studies of behavioral patterns in the bioethics field support the position that there is in fact no unified global field of bioethics. It seems that, even in English-speaking countries, bioethicists do not link to each other's websites as much as would be expected, do not cite each other as much as would be expected, and do not converge on the same books as much as would be expected if bioethics were truly a "global" field. These studies furthermore indicate that there are at least two types of disjunctions: 1) a geographical disjunction, or many depending on one's interpretation of the data, and 2) a disjunction between official bioethics and academic bioethics visible in the web linking analysis. If we had broadened our study to include non-English bioethics, we would undoubtedly have also found a linguistic disjunction. The most popular French and German bioethics books sold by Amazon in France and Germany are, for instance, even more dissimilar to the US or UK favorites in both topics and authors.[11]

Certain kinds of ethical ideas—philosophers call them "metaethical"—range beyond time and territory, thus allowing us to find coordinate meanings across communal and historic boundaries. For all their abstractness, they facilitate moral thinking about actual events and issues, or what is called "normative ethics." Experience reveals an interplay between actual events and abstract ideas or, as the late Harvard philosopher John Rawls called it, "reflexive equilibrium." Utility, duty, and virtue, for example, are found in Plato's *Republic* and in Aristotle's *Ethics* and *Politics*. Nor are these ideas absent from non-Western traditions, Confucian and Buddhist, for example. Indeed, this connectivity is what makes the study of diverse moral locations salient: new "content," perhaps, but "big" ideas, as some would have it. Ethics is an historical discipline. The contemporary emerges from but does not replace the classical.

Moral universals, over time, evolve in the face of different problems and issues. John Dewey remarked, for example, that we do not resolve moral conflicts, "we outgrow them." Temperament may lead some to stay with the "big" ideas of which events in the world are but instances. Others may build ethics upon the actual moral puzzles generated by the specific instance. There is neither reason nor need to settle the argument between the "hedgehog" and the "fox."[12] Ultimately, the concreteness of the moral problem, however situated and interpreted, is inescapable. Interpretation and redefinition are likewise inescapable.

DOING ETHICS IN A TIME OF TERRORISM

Terrorism today has features that we have never before encountered. The size and pace of things are different. We face the threat of "weapons of mass destruction." We can let loose powers that can destroy whole cities and make the land beneath and around them uninhabitable for generations. We can change the face of the planet itself. With genetically altered infectious agents or nuclear radiation, we can change the nature and number of its inhabitants; indeed, the human species itself. Food, air, and water supply become differently vulnerable.

Capability generates choices and thus gives rise to problems of good and evil. New capabilities thus force new choices. For example, a once clear distinction between combatant and noncombatant vanishes. Novel calculations of cost and benefit change the moral meanings of values like beneficence and harm. Terrorism is also a fact of the mind and spirit, a fact of culture and faith. With nuclear weaponry and genetic engineering, it is little wonder that apocalyptic thinking becomes a temptation. In religious terms, this world is surrendered to death. The next world waits. Islamists reinterpret suicide as martyrdom. Christian literalists read both natural cataclysm and intentional catastrophe as signs of the "end-time" forecast in Revelation.

> I heard, as it were the noise of thunder, one of the four beasts saying, come and see. And I saw, and behold a *white horse*: and he that sat on him had a bow; and a crown was given unto him: and he went forth conquering, and to conquer. . . . I heard the second beast say, come and see. And there went out another *horse that was red*: and power was given to him that sat thereon to take peace from the earth, and that they should kill one another: and there was given unto him a great sword. . . . And . . . I heard the third beast say, come and see. And I beheld, and lo a *black horse;* and he that sat on him had a pair of balances in his hand. . . . I heard the voice of the fourth beast say, come and see. And I looked, and behold a *pale horse*: and his name that sat on him was Death, and Hell followed with him. And power was given unto them over the fourth part of the earth, to kill with sword, and with hunger, and with death, and with the beasts of the earth.[13]

Both Islamist and Christian literalists move from imagery to conduct. Nor does secular culture escape the apocalyptic effect. Given 9/11, the Oklahoma bombing, Chernobyl, pandemic flu, SARS, and other catastrophes yet to come, both religious mythos and existential psychology erect their own realities. Developments in science and technology add a note of realism to the apocalyptic effect. In turn, the media reflect these developments outward to a public that is ready to believe. Thus,

- In 2000, Australian researchers genetically engineered a strain of mousepox virus in a way that inadvertently increased its virulence. At the time, publication of their findings was met with harsh criticism. This mousepox research and associated criticism were raised again in 2002 during additional debates on science and security.

- In July 2002, researchers at the State University of New York at Stony Brook revealed that they had successfully created infectious poliovirus from artificially engineered DNA sequences. Some observers saw open publication of their achievement in the journal *Science* as enabling the proliferation of a methodology with high BW potential.
- Researchers at the University of Pittsburgh identified key proteins in variola (smallpox) that contribute to the virus's virulence and demonstrated how to synthesize the virulence gene via genetic modification of smallpox's less deadly cousin vaccinia. The published report was the subject of a highly publicized news article that questioned the value of publishing discoveries that might aid bioterrorists.
- Researchers at the University of Pennsylvania successfully developed a hybrid virus composed of an HIV core surrounded by the surface proteins of ebola. This new virus was capable of infecting lung tissue, potentially enabling aerosol delivery, and could facilitate the expression of foreign genes in infected cells. The published findings arguably provided a roadmap to engineering of a viral vector capable of efficiently delivering bioregulatory agents.
- Researchers in Germany reported the creation of a DNA-based system for performing reverse genetics studies on the ebola virus. This system introduced the possibility of reconstituting live ebola virus from DNA in the absence of a viral sample. Other researchers expressed concern that this information could lead to the artificial synthesis of the virus, increasing the potential for agent proliferation, as DNA can be more safely transferred than viral samples.[14]

The modern experience sets the requirements of an ethical inquiry into the terrorist event. The size and pace of things, the evolution of science and technology, the move of culture and community into a time of terrorism—these pose questions of good and evil and, more likely, of choices between greater and lesser evils. Our inherited moral wisdom, no doubt, grounds contemporary moral inquiry in a usable past. It leaves us with the task of adapting that past to the world we are in and of creating a new moral past for those who will come after us without accepting the apocalyptic invitation.

NOTES

1. *From Clinic to Classroom: Medical Ethics and Moral Education*, Howard B. Radest, Praeger, Westport, CT, 2000.
2. "Oh, the Water . . . It Stoned Me to My Soul." *Newsletter*, University of Minnesota Center, Summer 2006.

3. We recognize this distinction when we identify clinical and organizational ethics as different subdisciplines. We give it operational meaning when we note that in dealing with access to health care we assign different moral status and duty to the "bedside" and to the institution. Thus, "rationing at the bedside" is regarded as morally questionable while failure to ration scarce resources fairly is regarded as moral abdication by professional communities and caregiving institutions.

4. The common-sense distinction between "natural" and "man-made" is a choice of convenience. In fact, the things we humans make and do are no more and no less natural than flood or hurricane or earthquake. But for my purposes, the common-sense distinction is useful even if misleading.

5. *The Smallpox Vaccination Program: Public Health in an Age of Terrorism*, Institute of Medicine, The National Academies Press, Washington, DC, 2005.

6. "Study Links Tropical Ocean Warming to Greenhouse Gases," Andrew C. Revkin, *NYT*, 9/12/06. The study was published online in The Proceedings of the National Academy of Sciences, 9/11/06.

7. "After the Tsunami—Facing the Public Health Challenges," Michael Van-Rooyen and Jennifer Leaning, *NEJM*, 352, 5, 2/3/05, pp. 435–38.

8. *Poetry and Imagination*, Ralph Waldo Emerson, 1872.

9. In 1971, Van Rensselaer Potter invented "bioethics" to refer to a field of ethical inquiry "devoted to human survival and an improved quality of life." [*Bioethics: Bridge to the Future*, Englewood Cliffs, NJ: Prentice-Hall]. Over time, the term came to include the moral problems posed by the life sciences—biology, medicine—and some aspects of the social sciences—the ethical dimensions of environmental and population studies, etc. As I reflected on ethics, catastrophe, and terrorism, I found that "bioethics," while not entirely satisfactory, could be expanded still further. Given the directions in which it has evolved, it captures or could capture most of what I was thinking about. In this I was following the lead of Daniel Callahan, who identified "two kinds of fundamental questions for bioethics to explore: First, what kind of medicine and health care, what kind of stance toward nature and our environment, do we need for the kind of society we want? The second question reverses the first: What kind of a society ought we to want in order that the life sciences will be encouraged and helped to make their best contribution to human welfare?"

"Bioethics" in the *Encyclopedia of Bioethics*, Rev. Ed., Macmillan, New York, 1995, p. 255.

10. *Principles of Biomedical Ethics*, Fourth Edition, Tom L. Beauchamp and James F. Childress, Oxford University Press, New York, 1994. For example, on page 37, they write,

> We defend what has sometimes been called the *four principles approach* to biomedical ethics, and also called, somewhat disparagingly, *principlism*. These principles initially derive from considered judgments in the common morality and the medical tradition. . . . For example, the principle of beneficence derives, in part, from long-standing, professional role obligations in medicine to provide medical benefits to patients. . . . Both the set of principles and the content ascribed to the principles are based on our attempt to put the common morality as a whole into a coherent package.

11. "Global Bioethics—Myth or Reality?" Soren Holm and Bryn Williams-Jones, *BioMed Central Medical Ethics* 10, 09/06/06, pp. 21–22.

12. In *The Hedgehog and the Fox* (New York, Simon & Schuster, 1953), Isaiah Berlin writes,

> There is a line among the fragments of the Greek poet Archilochus which says: "The fox knows many things, but the hedgehog knows one big thing". . . taken figuratively, the words can be made to yield a sense in which they mark one of the deepest differences which divide writers and thinkers, and, it may be, human beings in general. For there exists a great chasm between those, on one side, who relate everything to a single central vision, one system less or more coherent or articulate, in terms of which they understand, think and feel—a single, universal, organizing principle in terms of which alone all that they are and say has significance—and, on the other side, those who pursue many ends, often unrelated and even contradictory, connected, if at all, only in some *de facto* way, for some psychological or physiological cause, related by no moral or aesthetic principle; these last lead lives, perform acts, and entertain ideas that are centrifugal rather than centripetal, their thought is scattered or diffused, moving on many levels, seizing upon the essence of a vast variety of experiences and objects for what they are in themselves, without consciously or unconsciously, seeking to fit them into, or exclude them from, any one unchanging, all.

13. Revelation, chapter 6, verses 1 to 8.

14. "Intelligence Support to the Life Science Community: Mitigating Threats from Bioterrorism," James B. Petro, Joint Military Intelligence College, 2004.

3

The Law

SHAKESPEARE TO THE CONTRARY: WE CAN'T KILL ALL THE LAWYERS—NOR SHOULD WE!

Americans have a love/hate relationship with law and lawyers. Mixing piety and pragmatism, we use the law when in trouble, break it when it suits us, and honor it when it's threatened. We are a litigious people. We live in a country with more lawyers and more prisoners per capita than in any other industrialized country in the world. We stretch the law when dealing with things like speed limits and tax returns. But, when acts are seen to offend "public decency" (i.e., sexual behavior), we grow puritanical. Law becomes morality's executioner.

We connect law and ethics, sometimes as if law embodied ethical principles, at other times as if ethics was simply subsumed under law. The *social contract* tradition, on which we drew at the founding of our country (e.g., Hobbes, Locke, Hume, and Rousseau), mixed the two, concerned as they were with how people were governed and with how they could govern themselves. Tutored by the Enlightenment, Franklin, Jefferson, and Madison applied notions of natural law and social contract to justify revolution against church and monarch and to provide reason's basis for the new republic.

Tutored as well by Roman notions of civil (and "civilized") society and by Scripture's moral legalism, the founders understood *contract* as the "plain common sense" of the matter. Thus, they appealed to the British king in the name of the rights of Englishmen. Rejected by him, the Declaration of Independence appealed in the name of liberty, equality, and opportunity to a universal contract, as it were.

Since most of the founders were lawyers, as are most legislators to this day, they were already disposed to mix ethics and law. As American society evolved, it reflected this founding impulse. Indeed, it is typical of us, when dealing with ethical issues, to couch both problem and solution in legalistic terms. Of course, we have had ample reminders of immoral law. Injustice was surely exhibited in the constitutional provisions for dealing with slavery. The inferior and dependent status of women was shown in everything from denying their right to vote to denying their right to dispose of property. Yet the habit of turning ethics into law and vice versa continues to this day.

Taming law by ideal is no easy task. A single document like our Constitution, *pace* "strict constructionists," could not provide for the myriad details of interpersonal relationships. Nor could it accommodate the needs of an unimagined industrial and commercial society. Trying to bring order to an ever more complex federal system with multiple jurisdictions, each with its own history, territory, and constituency, is yet another constitutional puzzle. "Common law" traditions inherited from Great Britain were thus essential.[1] Cases, one by one, built a legal canon to which we could refer with some confidence in the law's stability, if not coherence. Thus, the role of precedent and *stare decisis*.

Given our roots in natural law, social contract, and common law, normative and descriptive notions were interwoven. Typically, Americans appeal to moral law—a "higher law" as we sometimes claim—against the law. To that end, the Supreme Court has become our paradigmatic institution. Despite occasions of dismay—Dred Scott in the nineteenth century, the abortion and civil rights controversies in the twentieth century, the Bush election in 2000 as the twenty-first century dawned—the Court enjoys near sacred status. For example, almost one hundred years later, Franklin Delano Roosevelt's attempt to "pack the court" is still condemned in moralistic if not in quasi-religious terms. It's a sure bet, however, that most of us recall the phrase but have little knowledge of the facts of the matter. Tellingly, few think to challenge the notion of having the tiniest of minorities—nine justices—resolve the weightiest issues of a democracy with 300 million citizens.

Nothing exhibits our complicated love affair with the law more than the Declaration of Independence, the Constitution, and the Bill of Rights. We treat them with the same reverence—and the same skepticism—that others attach to gods, idols, and monarchs. At the same time, we are hard-pressed to describe their contents. For example, when rights like religious freedom or free speech or due process are detached from these documents, we are as likely to reject as to applaud them. We are annoyed when rights are extended to less than popular causes or to "troublesome" minorities like "gays."

Iraq II and 9/11 have radically unsettled our idealization of the founding genius of the Republic. As Edward Lazarus writes,

> We are now engaged in a bitter debate over the constitutional framework within which the struggle against global terrorism must be fought. And that debate . . . encompasses at least three independent crosscurrents. First, there is a reasonably familiar tug-of-war between civil libertarians and post-9/11 "terror-hawks" over how much individual liberty and privacy ought to be sacrificed in order to better safeguard the country from future attacks. Second, there is a somewhat less familiar dispute over the power of the President to act independently from, or even override, the views of Congress in taking countermeasures against terrorist threats. And, third, there is a frequently ignored battle over how much the public is entitled to know about how the so-called war against terror is being conducted, so that the electorate can hold its public officials accountable for the policies they have chosen to pursue.[2]

Today, we encounter novel issues of the good, the lawful, and the constitutional, and the conflicts between them. We struggle with the problematic of fitting care and cure into contexts whose history and focus are elsewhere (i.e., on military and security priorities). At the same time, we are born, we suffer, and we die. Social realities and existential tensions meet in an uncomfortable struggle to accommodate the needs of intimacy and citizenship. So, it is not surprising that ethics must find its way in the midst of a constitutional controversy over the nature and uses of law in a democratic state living through a time of terrorism.

In order to exhibit this struggle, let us take a selective look at three legal moments: The USA PATRIOT Act and its amendments, the "police power," and the Model States Emergency Health Powers Act. Taken separately, each makes the case for necessary coercion in order to deal with catastrophic events. Taken together, they reveal a pattern that threatens the assumptions, values, and purposes of a free society.

THE PATRIOT ACT[3]

Those of us who do bioethics in hospital ethics committees or in the classroom focus on a familiar set of issues: autonomy, the right to refuse or withdraw treatment, informed consent, confidentiality, and privacy. Of course, we cannot avoid issues where bioethics and public policy meet; for example, abortion rights, access to health care, genetic "engineering," and so on. Always in the background are gender, race, and poverty. We are influenced too by religious values; we encounter minority mistrust of authority. When we add pandemic and environmental damage, the scope of bioethics widens still more. And, with the shifting dynamics of a "time of terrorism," it becomes impossible to isolate bioethics from the politics and economics of national security.

Within a few months of 9/11, the PATRIOT Act [2001] was voted into law by a nearly unanimous and bipartisan vote of the Congress. It was applauded by most of us as a good and necessary response to terrorism. Of course, the text nodded to civil liberties, due process, and the separation of powers. However, this seemed rhetorical piety rather than commitment to constitutional values, and subsequent practices verify that conclusion. Thus, as recently as October 2008, Attorney General Michael Mukasey,

> issued new guidelines for the FBI that permit agents to use a range of intrusive techniques to gather information on Americans—even when there is no clear basis for suspecting wrongdoing. Under the new rules, agents may engage in lengthy physical surveillance, covertly infiltrate lawful groups, or conduct pretext interviews in which agents lie about their identities while questioning a subject's neighbors, friends or work colleagues based merely on a generalized "threat." The new rules also allow the bureau to use these techniques on people identified in part by their race or religion and without requiring even minimal evidence of criminal activity.[4]

In short, the "imperial presidency," decades in the making, has reached new levels of unchecked authority.

There are provisions in the act that are useful, although most of them could have been achieved with fewer threats to the Constitution. In practice, the act subverts civil liberties and due process and not just for "nonstate combatants" or terrorists. As Richard Falk sums it up,

> The specific effects on human rights are . . . reflections of deficiencies in the human rights culture of the United States, and to a lesser extent in other countries. This is a large subject by itself, and can be encompassed by the rapid and uncritical omnibus legislation known as "The USA Patriot Act," which empowered the government to do in the name of anti-terrorism a series of previously prohibited activities intruding on the privacy and liberties of citizens and even more so, non-citizens . . . there were grounds for tightening security at the expense of rights in the light of the severe threats to fundamental security posed after September 11, but such initiatives could have been mainly taken on the basis of pre-existing legislation and carefully crafted supplemental laws.[5]

Tension between liberty and security is not unknown to us. In crisis—real or imagined—that tension is typically resolved, temporarily at least, in favor of security; for example, John Adams and the Alien and Sedition Acts, Lincoln and the suspension of habeas corpus, the Sedition Act of 1918 during and after World War I, Franklin Roosevelt's internment of West Coast Japanese in World War II, the Alien Registration Act (Smith Act, 1940) and the Internal Security Act (McCarran, 1950) during the Cold War. However, the historic record does not quite succeed as precedent for the PATRIOT Act. For example, reference to Lincoln's suspension of habeas corpus fails to note that the Congress was not in session and would not be for months and that Richmond, the Confederate capital and its military, were within one hundred miles of a chaotic and poorly defended Washington. The 1918 Sedition Act was enacted as the United States entered World War I. Despite that, the vote was not nearly as unanimous as the vote on the PATRIOT Act.[6] Indeed, the Sedition Act was repealed less than three years after its passage. Typically, these statutes ended when the real or perceived justification vanished. But a "war on terror" is easily made permanent. It has no intelligible end point.

The continuing shock of 9/11 explains our acceptance of the "war" metaphor. Worldwide terrorist events give it credibility. To name a few: the first Bali bombing (2002), the Riyadh compound bombings (2003), the Madrid train bombings, the Al-Khobar massacres, and the Jakarta embassy bombing (2004), the first and second London bombings, the Amman bombings, and the second Bali bombings (2005), the Mumbai train bombings and the transatlantic aircraft plot (2006). At the same time, except for 9/11 and the anthrax incidents, between 2001 and the renewal of the amended PATRIOT Act in 2006, there were no terrorist attacks in the United States.

In the climate of 9/11, it is difficult to challenge the move toward the "security" state and the laws that institutionalize it. Disenchantment with Iraq II does not affect that move. Indeed, a major complaint against Iraq II is that it misdirects our efforts to combat terrorism. In all probability, with a new administration in 2009, attention will shift to Afghanistan and its neighbors. But whether the power and influence of the PATRIOT Act will vanish remains an open question. Bioethical values are surely compromised. Autonomy becomes problematic. Justice becomes problematic, too. Nonmalificence yields to the needs of attack and defense. The debates about torture—"extreme interrogation techniques" is the government's euphemism—and about the indefinite confinement of "terrorists" illustrate an emerging pattern of widespread accommodation to what has historically been regarded as both illegal and immoral. As the *British Medical Journal* reported,

> Harsh treatment in the US detention camp at Guantanamo Bay has had profound effects on the mental health of many of the detainees and constitutes a breach of their right to health, a joint report by five UN independent experts has concluded. "The treatment and conditions include the capture and transfer of detainees to an undisclosed overseas location, sensory deprivation and other abusive treatment during transfer; detention in cages without proper sanitation and exposure to extreme temperatures; minimal exercise and hygiene; systematic use of coercive interrogation techniques; and long period[s] of solitary confinement," it says. The report to the UN Human Rights Council is by the special rapporteurs on torture.[7]

Caregivers, attorneys, chaplains, the military itself, etc., find themselves serving as torture's helpers. Hunger strikes and forced feeding continue to be subjects of controversy.[8] The courts, including the Supreme Court, repeatedly call for habeas corpus and due process. The executive response is excuse and delay that by now seems more like deliberate defiance than reflective need.

With these considerations in mind, we come directly to the PARIOT Act. Section 215 (2001) provides a relevant example. It "Authorizes the Director of the FBI (or designee) to apply for a court order requiring production of certain business records for foreign intelligence and international terrorism investigations." It "Requires the Attorney General to report to the House and Senate Intelligence and Judiciary Committees semi-annually."[9]

But Section 215 is not innocent. It allows federal investigators access to library and bookstore records of anyone connected to an investigation of international terrorism. The necessary warrant, when and if sought, is granted "in camera," (i.e., secretly) by the U.S. Foreign Intelligence Surveillance Court (FISA), whose deliberations are also secret. "Business records" are not defined. In effect, an investigator is authorized to conduct a nearly limitless search of the records of just about any individual or group including finances, travel logs, book purchases, video rentals, phone logs, health care, contributions, and contributors. The only requirement is a claim of "investigative necessity." The "in camera" provision has been interpreted to mean that institutions whose records are examined are forbidden to inform the person or persons that they were the objects of a search. An amendment [2006] made minor changes, calling for agreement from officials higher up in the chain of command. Thus, "*Requests for Sensitive Information Such as Library or Medical Records:* Without the personal approval of one of these three officials (FBI Director, Deputy Director, or Official-in-Charge of Intelligence), the 215 order for these sensitive categories of records may not be issued." Recently, even that oversight is eroded as new powers are vested in the executive branch.

Section 1013 provides for the support of public health and health care institutions. However, public health budgets, already miniscule, are now required to give priority to the new mission (i.e., to bioterrorism and national security). In adopting Section 1013, the "sense of the Senate" reads, in part,

> (2) The threat of a bioterrorist attack is still remote, but is increasing for a variety of reasons, including—
>
> (A) public pronouncements by Osama bin Laden that it is his religious duty to acquire weapons of mass destruction, including chemical and biological weapons;
>
> (B) the callous disregard for innocent human life as demonstrated by the terrorists' attacks of September 11, 2001;
>
> (C) the resources and motivation of known terrorists and their sponsors and supporters to use biological warfare;

(D) recent scientific and technological advances in agent delivery technology such as aerosolization that have made weaponization of certain germs much easier; and
(E) the increasing access to the technologies and expertise necessary to construct and deploy chemical and biological weapons of mass destruction.

HIPAA[10] regulations, developed over more than a decade of debate, were intended, among other things, to protect the confidentiality of medical records. However, in the following advisory published by The Center for Law and the Public's Health at Georgetown and Johns Hopkins universities, the influence of the PATRIOT Act is visible,

> ISSUE: Do the new federal health information privacy regulations [HIPAA] limit the disclosure of individually identifiable health information by covered entities to public health authorities pursuant to bioterrorism or other reporting requirements?
>
> RESPONSE: For the reasons set forth below, the HIPAA privacy regulations *do not substantially limit these disclosures. In fact, the HIPAA privacy regulations encourage and support the disclosure of individually-identifiable data without specific, informed consent for public health purposes.*[11]

In short, privacy, already a problem in a data-rich society, becomes even more problematic. A repeated pattern appears: the claim to protect liberty in theory and undercut it in practice. *1984*'s *newspeak* and *doublethink* are not far away. While the PATRIOT Act is only the most dubious moment in the struggle between community needs and individual conscience, other efforts have been less problematic.

POLICE POWER

Public health and clinical care live in the same moral neighborhood. They share the caregiving professions: physicians, nurses, social workers, researchers, and technicians. They also share moral values like distributive justice, autonomy, and beneficence. Unlike clinical care, however, public health engages populations and communities. Investigation, surveillance, and enforcement are among its tools. Nor is the military entirely absent, e.g., National Guard units are mobilized to deal with catastrophic events. Individuals may have their rights overridden where the public good demands. Of course, as rational moral agents in the midst of catastrophe, they should expect no less. So, in a democratic society, there is a permanent tension between coercion and liberty.

Public health uses a utilitarian ethic; that is, the "greatest good for the greatest number." This would seem a natural entry point for counterterrorism. Like public health, counterterrorism aims to sustain community against threat to its existence. But the rhetoric of warfare and the realities of tactics and strategy transform traditional community goals. An enemy is at work and must be defeated. In turn, national security reshapes the duties of professionals and the psyches of citizens. The unboundaried character of a "war on terrorism" invites anxiety and belligerence. Sooner or later, the public health mission is subverted.

Consider Homeland Security: an alert system that people ignore, airport security that fails to secure, seizure of suspects and other "persons of interest" using lists that have not been checked for errors. Clinical concerns, like the attempt at mass smallpox vaccination, mix public health preparedness and security requirements. Defeating an enemy at whatever cost becomes the guiding principle.

But, the situation is ambiguous. For all that we are said to be "at war," we are encouraged not to let terrorism change the way we live. Terrorist attacks are episodic and distant. Thus far, since 9/11 and anthrax, there have been no such attacks in the United States. In fact, the enemy is not some grand conspiracy but more likely small groups of irregulars, some well trained, some not, appearing out of the shadow world and disappearing back into it.

Whatever its other purposes, the PATRIOT Act exploits the ambiguity of being and not being at war, attempts to dissolve anxiety into the simplicity of either/or. It is a flawed, even dangerous, instrument. By contrast, "police power" is the traditional justification of public health's use of coercion. It relies on law, the courts, professional ethics, and history to secure the safety and welfare of its citizens. It roots its legitimacy in multiple sovereignties—states, municipalities, and federal government—providing, as it were, another form of "checks and balances." The first public health ordinances were enacted by Boston in 1647 and by New York in 1663. With the establishment of the Republic and the adoption of the Tenth Amendment to the Constitution, powers not specifically delegated to the federal government were reserved to the states that, in turn, were also sovereign within their jurisdictions.

Among the first judicial references to the police powers was Chief Justice Marshall's opinion in an 1824 case. He wrote, "the immense mass of legislation which embraces everything within the territory of a State, not surrendered to the general government. . . . Inspection laws, quarantine laws, health laws of every description, as well as laws for regulating the internal commerce of a State."[12]

The classic precedent for police powers was and still is *Jacobson v. Massachusetts*, decided by the Supreme Court in 1905.

> In June 1894, the Commonwealth of Massachusetts enacted a law that allowed municipalities to order the compulsory vaccination of its residents during disease outbreaks. When the Boston smallpox epidemic that began in May 1901 spread to surrounding towns, the Cambridge Board of Health in February 1902 ordered its residents who had not received the smallpox vaccine since March 1897 to be vaccinated. Jacobson, the minister of the Swedish Evangelical Lutheran Church in Cambridge, had been vaccinated against smallpox as a child and had experienced a serious reaction to the vaccine. Jacobson refused to comply with the Board of Health's vaccination order. Charged with violating the law, Jacobson plead not guilty in the municipal court, but was eventually convicted and fined $5. After the Massachusetts Supreme Court upheld the lower court's decision, Jacobson appealed his case to the US Supreme Court.[13]

In his brief, Jacobson had claimed that the State had abused its police power and that the statute mandating vaccination was "socialist." Before the Supreme Court he claimed that his due process rights under the Fourteenth Amendment had been violated. In upholding the lower courts and the Massachusetts' Supreme Court decision against Jacobson, Justice Harlan wrote,

> The authority of the State to enact this statute is to be referred to what is commonly called the *police power*. . . . Although this court has refrained from any attempt to define the limits of that power, yet it has distinctly recognized the authority of a State to enact quarantine laws and "health laws of every description." According to settled principles, the *police power* of a State must be held to embrace, at least, such reasonable regulations established directly by legislative enactment as will protect the public health and the public safety. . . . [T]he liberty secured by the *Constitution of the United States* to every person within its jurisdiction does not import an absolute right in each person to be, at all times and in all circumstances, wholly freed from restraint. There are manifold restraints to which every person is necessarily subject for the common good. . . . This court has more than once recognized it as a fundamental principle that "persons and property are subjected to all kinds of restraints and burdens, in order to secure the general comfort, health, and prosperity of the State." Upon the principle of self-defense, of paramount necessity, a community has the right to protect itself against an epidemic of disease which threatens the safety of its members.[14]

While practice, statute, and judicial decision have, by and large, focused on the powers of states and localities for dealing with public health issues, a federal role has also developed. Its justification is the "commerce clause" of the Constitution. Article I, Section 8, reads in part: "The Congress shall have the power to lay and collect taxes . . . *provide for the common defense and general welfare of the United States* . . . to regulate commerce with foreign nations and among the several states." As interpreted by the courts, the commerce clause is the source of an indefinitely large number of federal powers in peacetime. It provides legal authority for federal action in health care, education, transportation, as well as in the more obvious matters of trade, business, and labor. Indeed, with the regionalization and nationalization of the country under modern conditions, the phrases "the common defense and general welfare" and "among the several states" appear to justify a larger and larger role for the federal government.

Taken together, the interpretation of the commerce clause and the sovereign's police powers would appear to offer sufficient sanction for responding to the needs of counterterrorism. However, such an interpretation also opens the door to nearly indefinite extension of federal powers in a time of mortal threat. Even so nebulous a notion as a "war on terror" could be sanctioned. Against the "police power" so interpreted, civil liberties and rights are a weak protection not merely in the counsels of government but in the homes and streets of the community itself. On the other hand, the tradition of judicial review and legislative oversight evident in the record of the police power is far stronger than the meager provisions of the PATRIOT Act. No doubt imperfect, the "police power" is more promising. On the other hand, as with other Supreme Court decisions, it could also be more threatening. The PATRIOT Act, after all, can be repealed in a representative government. Court decisions are resistant to legislation and, given the separation of powers, are authorized to be so.

EMERGENCY POWERS

If the PATRIOT Act empowers the national executive, the newly established Department of Homeland Security is its institutional base. By contrast, the Model State Emergency Health Powers Act [MSEHPA] is an effort to bring public health law up-to-date in a time of terrorism within existing institutional structures. Its context is the public health legal tradition. *Jacobson v. Massachusetts* remains its source along with nearly two centuries of legal precedent. Like the PATRIOT Act and the police power, the Model Act recognizes that crises emerge quickly, cross national, state, and local boundaries, cannot wait upon the time-consuming processes of legislative and judicial practice, and must avoid the give and get of interest group political negotiation. From Jacobson on, the expansion of police powers is but "necessity" writ large.

As the principle convener of the task force that drafted MSEHPA, Lawrence Gostin wrote, "The law-reform process took on new urgency after the terrorist attacks of late 2001. In response, the CLPH (Center for Law and Public Health) drafted MSEHPA at the request of the CDC."[15] He and his colleague, James Hodge, sum up the act's provisions:

Sets a high threshold definition of what constitutes a "public health emergency" [Article I];

Requires the development of a comprehensive public health emergency response plan [Article II];

Authorizes the collection of data and records and access to communications to facilitate the early detection of a health emergency [Article III];

Vests the power to declare a public health emergency in the state governor, subject to appropriate legislative and judicial checks and balances [Article IV];

Grants state and local public health officials the authority to use and appropriate property to care for patients, destroy dangerous or contaminated materials, and implement safe handling procedures for the disposal of human remains or infectious wastes [Article V];

Authorizes officials to care for and treat ill or exposed persons, to separate affected individuals from the population at large to prevent further transmission [Article VI];

Requires public health authorities to inform the population of public health threats [Article VII];

Authorizes the governor to allocate state finances as needed during an emergency, and creates limited immunities for some state and private actors from future legal causes of action [Article VIII].[16]

The act focuses on the responsibilities of state government. However, as with catastrophes like Katrina and the anthrax events, it recognizes the need to cross jurisdictions. It also tries to provide for public pressure that may well force a reluctant governor or president to act despite precedent, political risk, and the force of jurisdictional prerogative.

The powers delegated to state governors are among the act's more controversial provisions. Following a declaration of emergency, a governor may "Suspend the provisions of any regulatory statute prescribing procedures for conducting State business, or the orders, rules and regulations of any State agency, to the extent that strict compliance with the same would prevent, hinder, or delay necessary action (including emergency purchases) by the public health authority." He or she may "mobilize all or any part of the organized militia into service of the State." He or she may "seek aid from the federal government in accordance with federal programs or requirements."[17]

It would be surprising indeed if the Model Act were not criticized for violating civil liberties and constitutional rights. George Annas, for example, writes,

> Although the revised act [December 21, 2001] can be viewed as a modest improvement [over the original draft], all the fundamental problems remain. Failure to comply with the orders of public health officials for examination or treatment is no longer a crime but results in isolation or quarantine. . . . Physicians and other health care providers can still be required "to assist" public

> health officials, but cooperation is now coerced as "a condition of licensure" instead of a legal requirement with criminal penalties for non-compliance.

Quarantine has been and remains among the more problematic public health powers legally and morally. Annas continues,

> Quarantine can be ordered when the person's refusal to be examined or tested "results in uncertainty regarding whether he or she has been exposed to or is infected with a contagious or possibly contagious disease or otherwise poses a danger to public health." This is no standard at all; it simply permits public health authorities to quarantine anyone who refuses to be examined or treated, for whatever reason, since all refusals will result in uncertainty. . . . These vague standards are especially troublesome because the act's incredible immunity provision remains unchanged. Thus, all state public health officials and all private companies and persons operating under their authority are granted immunity from liability for their actions (except for gross negligence or willful misconduct), even in the case of death or permanent injury.[18]

Despite criticism, the act has been widely adopted in whole or part and, typically, as an amendment to existing pubic health statutes. Troubling is the fact that many state legislatures have acted on it without significant public notice or debate. As of 2006, thirty-eight states and the District of Columbia had incorporated most of the provisions of MSEHPA.[19]

Gostin is sensitive to the need for public participation, reminding us that, "The act was written in collaboration with members of national organizations representing governors, legislators, public health commissions, and attorneys general. There was also an extensive consultative process involving the major stakeholders such as businesses, public health and civil liberties organizations, scholars, and practitioners."[20] Nor is he indifferent to the tension between civil liberties and security. For example, Article V, Section 504 of the act provides that public health authorities have the power "to order the disposal of any human remains of a person who has died of a contagious disease through burial or cremation within twenty-four (24) hours after death." But the act cautions, "To the extent possible, religious, cultural, family, and individual beliefs of the deceased person or his or her family shall be considered when disposing of any human remains." When challenged, Gostin notes that the act provides for the automatic termination of a state of emergency after thirty days unless specifically renewed by the governor. It further provides that after sixty days, a majority of both chambers of a state legislature can overrule the governor and declare the state of emergency ended.

In justifying his work, Gostin points out that individualism is not the only moral theme of American culture. A "communitarian" tradition is part of our history, too. Concern for the general welfare, while no doubt muted in today's America, is nevertheless a genuine good. He is not blind to First

Amendment critiques or states' rights claims. As he puts it, "The balance between individual interests and common goods needs to be recalibrated in an age of terrorism." After all, the same Constitution that establishes civil rights and liberties is introduced by a communal statement: "We the people, in order to form a more perfect union."

EXPANDING AGENDA

Terrorism has expanded and to no little extent distorted the bioethics agenda, forced us to amend our epistemology, and introduced new players or old players in new roles into the field. It has created new victims and afflicted them with new forms of suffering, not least of all the emotional suffering of a time of terrorism where threat does not vanish. Thus, the increase of what the theologian calls "existential anxiety" and for not a few what psychiatrists call "posttraumatic stress disorder." Of course, nature's cataclysm, human error, and the human condition itself introduce us to disaster and suffering often enough. But, things are different since 9/11. Hence the question: what has terrorism done to the helping professions and to their patients, to the practices of care and cure, and to the law and the military and ultimately to the wounded community and its inhabitants?

We need not impugn the motives of those who have advanced and those who have criticized the law's response to terrorism and to catastrophic events. Of course, the PATRIOT Act and the Emergency Health Powers Act look to different ends and exhibit different values. The latter aims to strengthen existing structures; the former, to replace them. Both, however, are moved by the threats, actual and imagined, to the public welfare. However different, their advocates conclude that states and municipalities have become incompetent jurisdictions and that traditional rights and liberties can be dangerous to survival in a time of terror.

Yet, we should remember that the "police power" also entailed an erosion of personal rights and liberties, a thought implicit in Annas's critique of MSEHPA. The issue is as old as the Republic, the tension when in crisis between liberty and security, between autonomy and authority. It is, of course, a matter of power and of those in power. In short, the law both protects and jeopardizes due process and civil liberty. Much depends on who reads the law, how it is read, when it is read, and by whom it is administered. Safeguards against the overreaching executive face an age-old dilemma, "who guards the guardians." Both the PATRIOT Act and MSEHPA are bureaucratically driven. The rule and character of the expert and of expert authority become central problems of democratic society. With these concerns in mind, I turn to consideration of instances of disaster, natural or man-made, and their moral dimensions.

NOTES

1. "Common law is based largely on case law, i.e., on court decisions. It began in the United Kingdom hundreds of years ago and developed from the rules and principles that judges traditionally followed in deciding court cases. Judges based their decisions on legal precedents—that is, on earlier court rulings in similar cases. But judges could expand precedents to make them suit particular cases. They could also overrule (reject) any precedents that they considered to be in error or outdated. In this way, judges changed many laws over the years. Common law thus came to be law made by judges." *World Book Encyclopedia*, 2004.

2. "How Has 9/11 Affected American Constitutional Law? The Three Intersecting Cross-Currents that Have Affected Liberty, Security, and Government Accountability," Edward Lazarus, *Find Law*, 9/15/06.

3. The Uniting and Strengthening America by Providing Appropriate Tools Required to Intercept and Obstruct Terrorism Act of 2001 (Public Law 107-56), commonly known as the PATRIOT Act, was signed into law by President George W. Bush on October 26, 2001. President Bush signed its amended form on March 9, 2006.

4. "Another Invitation to Abuse,"Editorial, *NYT*, 10/19/08.

5. Richard Falk, "Human Rights, A Descending Spiral," in *Human Rights in the 'War on Terror,'* Richard Ashby Wilson, editor, Cambridge University Press, New York, 2005, p. 232.

6. The 2001 act passed in the Senate by a vote of 98 to 1, and in the House by a vote of 357 to 66. It was renewed on March 2, 2006, with a vote of 89 to 11 in the Senate and on March 7, 280 to 138 in the House.

7. "Guantanamo Breaches Right to Health, Says UN," John Zarocostas, *BMJ*, 333, 09/30/06, p. 670.

8. "Glimpses of Guantanamo—Medical Ethics and the War on Terror," Susan Okie, MD, *NEJM*, Vol 353, 24, 12/15/05, pp. 2529–2534; Physicians for Human Rights, Report on U.S. Torture, 2005. The American Medical Association issued the following statement,

The AMA has shared with U.S. military officials its position on hunger strikes or feeding individuals against their will. Specifically, the AMA endorses the World Medical Association's Declaration of Tokyo, which states:

> Where a prisoner refuses nourishment and is considered by the physician as capable of forming an unimpaired and rational judgment concerning the consequences of such a voluntary refusal of nourishment, he or she shall not be fed artificially. The decision as to the capacity of the prisoner to form such a judgment should be confirmed by at least one other independent physician.

The American Medical Association is the largest professional organization of physicians in the United States; however, we are not a regulatory or licensing agency. Over the past year, the AMA has met with the Department of Defense to voice our concerns, provide them with relevant policies, and offer our expertise with the goal of ensuring that U.S. policies on detainee treatment comport with ethical standards of medicine. The AMA will continue to advocate for treatment of all detainees in U.S. custody to be in accordance with our Code of Medical Ethics and the Geneva

Conventions. Our physician colleagues in the military, many of whom are placed in difficult, sometimes dangerous situations, deserve nothing less. [March 10, 2006]

9. "Bill Summary & Status for the 107th Congress: H.R.3162." It became Public Law No: 107-56.

10. "In the United States, the *Health Insurance Portability and Accountability Act* (HIPAA) of 1996 took effect early in 2004 after extensive planning and discussion. The new regulations provide protection for the privacy of certain individually identifiabie health data, referred to as protected health information. The privacy rules permit disclosures without individual authorization to public health authorities authorized by law to collect or receive the information for the purpose of preventing or controlling disease, injury, or disability, including public health practice activities such as surveillance."

"Ethical Issues in Epidemiologic Research and public Health Practice," Steven S. Coughlin, *Emerging Themes in Epidemiology*, 2006, 3:16.

11. "Bioterrorism Surveillance under HIPAA's Public Health Exception," James G. Hodge, Jr., J.D., LL.M., Deputy Director, *Center for Law and the Public's Health*, 02/20/03. Emphasis added.

12. *Gibbons v. Ogden*, 22 US I, 87, 1824.

13. "Uses of *Jacobson v. Massachusetts* in the Age of Bioterror," D. George Joseph, *JAMA*, 290, 2003, 2331.

14. *Jacobson v. Massachusetts*, 197 US 1 [1905].

15. "Public Health Law in an Age of Terrorism: Rethinking Individual Rights and Common Goods. In Defense of a Model Act That Was Written to Bring Public Health Law into the Modern Age." Lawrence O. Gostin, *Health Affairs*, Volume 21:6, November/December 2002, pp. 82-83.

16. Citations and notes are from *Commentary on the Model State Emergency Health Powers Act*, Lawrence O. Gostin and James G. Hodge, Jr., The Turning Point, Public Health Statute Modernization Collaborative, 2002.

17. MSEHPA, Article IV, 403.

18. "Bioterrorism, Public Health, and Civil Liberties," George J. Annas, J.D., M.P.H., *N Engl J Med*, Vol. 346, No. 17, 04/25/02, pp. 1337-42.

The language of the Model Act on quarantine is instructive. For example, Article VI, Section 605 addresses quarantine and provides among other things,

> (a) Temporary isolation and quarantine without notice.
>
> (1) Authorization. The public health authority may temporarily isolate or quarantine an individual or groups of individuals through a written directive if delay in imposing the isolation or quarantine would significantly jeopardize the public health authority's ability to prevent or limit the transmission of a contagious or possibly contagious disease to others. . . .
>
> (b) Isolation or quarantine with notice.
>
> (1) Authorization. The public health authority may make a written petition to the trial court for an order authorizing the isolation or quarantine of an individual or groups of individuals.
>
> (4) (i) an order authorizing isolation or quarantine may do so for a period not to exceed thirty (30) days.
>
> (6) Continuances. . . . the public health authority may move to continue isolation or quarantine for additional periods not to exceed thirty (30) days each. . . .

(e) Court to appoint counsel and consolidate claims.

(1) Appointment. The court shall appoint counsel at state expense to represent individuals or groups of individuals who are or who are about to be isolated or quarantined pursuant to the provisions of this Act. . . . The public health authority must provide adequate means of communication between such individuals or groups and their counsel.

19. *Legislative Update,* Center for Law and the Public's Health, a federally funded project at Georgetown and Johns Hopkins universities.

20. Gostin, "Public Health Law in an Age of Terrorism," p. 83.

4

Katrina: Rehearsal for Terrorism

In America, even with our incommensurable memories of 9/11, we still do not have an exact human vocabulary for the loss of a city—our great iconic city, so graceful, livable, insular, self-delighted, eccentric, the one New Orleansians always said, with a wink, that care forgot and that sometimes, it might seem, forgot to care. Other peoples have experienced their cities' losses. Some bombed away (sometimes by us). Others, gone in the flood. Here now is one more tragedy that we thought, by some divinity's grace that didn't arrive, we'd miss. And our inept attempts at words run only to lists, costs, to assessing blame. It's like Hiroshima, a public official said. But no. It's not like anything. It's what it is. That's the hard part. He, with all of us, lacked the words. . . . Empathy is what we long for—not sadness for a house we own, or owned once—now swept away. . . . It's hard to make sense of this, we say. But it makes sense. Making sense just doesn't help.

—Richard Ford, *New York Times*[1]

HAS BIOETHICS FAILED?[2]

Katrina was terrifying, but it was not terrorism. It had its causes of course—some no doubt human—but it was not the work of an enemy unless nature itself be charged with hostility. Of course, Katrina had its villains, heroes, and fools, its violence, and, above all, its victims. But before turning to its story, Katrina—and it is not the only example—challenges the way we conceive bioethics. The discipline has evolved over several decades, but it remains rooted in a clinical and research environment. That environment, however, is changing. Experience itself is reperceived. Hence, my questions: What has terrorism done to our perceptions, feelings and judgments? How shall bioethics become adequate to political and social chaos and catastrophe?

Let me start with a bit of autobiography. More than two decades ago, I began to work in the field. Like so many others, almost without realizing its limitations, I learned to understand bioethics in clinical terms. My vocabulary was medical; indeed, it was only later that "medical ethics" became "biomedical ethics," a reminder of the discipline's other base in research and the sciences. The compound names thus clearly revealed their sources and history. Now, we rechristen it "bioethics." If the name is not merely nominal—and I think it is much more than that—it tells us that political, social, and cultural context is unavoidably causal and explanatory.

Earlier, my attention as a teacher and as a hospital ethics committee chair was on the sick and the dying and on those who tried to help them back to health or ease them less painfully from this life. The typical questions that concerned me had to do with how, where, and why treatment and treatment institutions had gone morally awry. Issues of social policy arose from the morally troubling responses to specific cases or—as the literature sometimes has it—to "classic" cases like Quinlan and Dax and Schiavo. But, in the forefront still was the relationship of doctor and patient. Gradually and belatedly, nurses acquired near equal status in our view of that relationship, but the individualism of that relationship did not change. Social issues remained derivative of my focus on the medically deprived and mistreated. Issues of religion, race, and gender appeared, too. These too were also focused on the patient, on access and its inadequacy, now complicated by culture. Only secondarily, so to speak, did I explore the import of the larger surround, like a market economy with its selling and buying of health care itself—the patient viewed as "consumer," and so on—and the consequent issues of distributive *injustice*. In short, my ethics was individualistic and medicalized, and I was not alone.

Two other agendas shaped my understanding of the move to biomedical ethics. The first, different from but closely related to the needs of the sick, was research and its issues: the limits of human experimentation, the exploitive behaviors of drug companies, the obligations, sometimes in conflict, to research "subjects" and to scientific inquiry. Here again, whatever their larger import, the focus was on care and cure, on individuals, now called "subjects," in the medical situation. In teaching, I invoked a bit of history, too. But, as typically presented in texts and journals, it corroborated a clinical pathway into the field. Nuremberg and Tuskegee, to name two iconic events of biomedical history, sanctioned my attentiveness to victims and their pathologies or to subjects and their moral rights. Nazism and racism, however, were only superficially addressed, a throwaway reference perhaps or an unspecific background footnote. Not to exaggerate the point, it was nevertheless true that the clinical environment was parochial, reflecting, no doubt, both a necessary prudence—pain didn't wait, time was always too short, and the agenda always too long—and the specialism that afflicts medicine and other social institutions in our technologized society.

The other thread was public health, the shift from individuals to populations.[3] Surprising myself when I reflect on it—I knew better—public health was a latecomer to my consciousness and it began to move me toward bioethics. I would dare the thought that most of us doing ethics in clinic, laboratory, or political lobby today followed a similar trajectory. Here my experience as a sometime social activist and no doubt by the fact that I had lived through the 1960s reminded me of an Aristotelian wisdom, that the human being is a social animal and that ethics and politics are inextricably interwoven. So to invoke the one is to invoke the other. To conceive the human being otherwise as the eighteenth century's creature of ego and desire connected to others by self-interest and sentiment is to commit a serious philosophic and psychological error.

With these shifting perspectives, another horizon came into view. The morally relevant scene is never really boundaried by the walls of the hospital, the classroom, or the laboratory. Indeed, health itself is a communal problem and its solution awaits a communal answer. The greater achievements of modern health care—decreased infant morality, longer life spans, active biographies over more and more decades of life—are the result of communal efforts with housing, sanitation, water supply, and diet far more than with the undoubted successes of doctoring and its individualized model.

And so, provoked by terrorism, I found my ethics making a perceptual, epistemic, and moral move toward history, culture, and society. Terrorism, today's preoccupation, stimulated an unavoidable consciousness of violence and hostility and their relevance to the bioethical scene. Its horizon expands not once but many times. Hence this second part of my essay looks to differing dimensions of care and cure in the move from individuals to populations and in particular, to populations living under threat, real or imagined. A caution, however: this does not signal desertion of persons in trouble but a reconsideration of how they got to the point of needing and benefiting from the ministrations of doctors, nurses, technicians, social workers, and chaplains; yes, and lawyers, business managers, bankers, politicians, and even ethicists. There are indeed a growing number of "strangers at the bedside." At the same time, the move from individuals to populations asks for reconsideration not only of those "done-to" but also of those "doing-for."

To be sure, individuals still inhabit the territories of bioethics, but moral adequacy commands attention to individuals in settings more encompassing, more natural, and more salient than clinic and laboratory, both of which are, as it were, usable but limited artificial habitats. Following the questions with which I opened this chapter, bioethics needs to accept an often unmanageable but unavoidable Aristotelian necessity, the undivided connection between ethics and politics. Of course, it was always there but unattended to, as it were. Hence, this exploration of the events—only some of them terrorist—that terrify us and the settings in which they happen, with which we try to cope, and from which we try to emerge. Katrina is such an event; indeed, in its own way a signal event and no doubt on its way to becoming a different kind of "classic" case.[4]

A DISASTER WAITING TO HAPPEN

Natural disasters kill thousands, destroy cities, and devastate environments. Sadly, they are unavoidable. I am reminded of tsunami and earthquake, fire and flood, of Pompeii and Mount St. Helens and Aceh. I am reminded too of terrorist events, some of which in their magnitude compete with our own—and our owned—9/11.[5] Katrina joins the list. It was indeed the "perfect storm," although, as we know, error and cupidity, joining nature, contributed in no little way to its outcomes. Two years later, its direct costs were estimated at $82 billion. How much that number will grow is still unknown. And three years later, New Orleans has yet to emerge fully from Katrina's damage and people's failure. Deaths exceeded 2,000, with others lost and uncounted. Some 90,000 square miles, the coastlines of three states—Alabama, Louisiana, and Mississippi—were devastated. Tens of thousands were displaced. Many dispersed across the United States never to return home.

In the beginning was the prediction.

> New Orleans is a disaster waiting to happen. The city lies below sea level, in a bowl bordered by levees that fend off Lake Pontchartrain to the north and the Mississippi River to the south and west. And because of a damning confluence of factors, the city is sinking further, putting it at increasing flood risk after even minor storms. The low-lying Mississippi Delta, which buffers the city from the gulf, is also rapidly disappearing. A year from now another 25 to 30 square miles of delta marsh—an area the size of Manhattan—will have vanished. An acre disappears every 24 minutes. Each loss gives a storm surge a clearer path to wash over the delta and pour into the bowl, trapping one million people inside and another million in surrounding communities. Extensive evacuation would be impossible because the surging water would cut off the few escape routes.[6]

And in the beginning were other priorities. The needs of commerce built the Mississippi River Gulf Outlet (MR-GO) in order to straighten out the course of the river and facilitate the movement of shipping into and out of the Gulf. The hubris of such a venture, surely a promise of trouble to come, is indeed a reminder of classic tragedy. As an advertisement once had it, "You can't fool mother nature." Heavy winds and storm surges breached its levees in more than twenty places. Budget cuts constrained the U.S. Army's Corps of Engineers, already limited by a narrowly mechanistic orientation, which had done as much as the money said they could do. So, the levees—built knowingly to withstand weaker storms—could not hold. Ultimately, nearly 80 percent of New Orleans was flooded. Little wonder that "roads became rivers." These were the markers of so many years of neglect, of so many poor choices made, of dangerous postponements made, and of dubious predictions made.[7]

With the storm only hours away, the National Weather Service warned,

> A most powerful hurricane with unprecedented strength . . . most of the area will be uninhabitable for weeks . . . perhaps longer. . . . At least one half of well-constructed homes will have roof and wall failure. . . . The majority of industrial buildings will become non-functional. . . . High rise office and apartment buildings will sway dangerously. . . . Airborne debris will be widespread. . . . Power outages will last for weeks. . . . The vast majority of native trees will be snapped or uprooted.[8]

But by then, it was too late to do anything but run.

WHERE ARE THE BUSES?

It wasn't the wind; it was the water—two feet deep in some places, nearly twenty in others. Four out of very five of the city's inhabitants, some 400,000 people, found safety elsewhere following the mayor's order of a mandatory evacuation on August 28th, one day before the hurricane arrived. The rest, more than 100,000, had to make do with emergency shelters and the roofs and attics of homes, the hospitals, the upper floors of hotels and offices. None of these "shelters" was particularly sheltering as the wind shook the buildings and the waters kept on rising.

Soon, electric power failed. With that, suffering and death increased. Against the city's torrid climate—the end of summer's unrelieved heat and humidity—air conditioning became unavailable except in some few buildings like the finer hotels that had their own emergency generators. Pumps couldn't work. Refrigeration stopped. Food and drinkable water became scarce. Most of the left-behind population remained calm. However, looting, that at first had the laudable if illegal purpose of finding food and drink in stores closed against the storm, soon included a criminal few in free-for-all raids on goods and goodies—including, notably, handguns—left unprotected by their owners and by the police as well. Here and there, shots were heard, but it wasn't clear what was being shot at and why the snipers were shooting.

The weakest and those trapped on lower floors of buildings or in poorly built houses died quickly enough, adding the smell of decaying corpses to the stench of unwashed bodies and the mounting heaps of garbage and debris. The scenes, broadcast live over national and international TV, looked like those shown when disasters strike in developing countries. But, given our wealth and technical know-how, these images were all the more shocking, unexpected, and demoralizing.

Offers of help came from the rest of the country and from abroad as well. Strangely, arrogantly perhaps, American pride perhaps, these latter offers were not accepted. Contributions to agencies like the Red Cross and the Salvation Army for hurricane relief soon exceeded a record $1 billion. But the city wasn't ready for rescue.

It was too late to do anything but run. But the 100,000 could not run. Who were they? No surprises here: the black, the poor, the sick, and the old. In New Orleans before Katrina, 12 percent of the people were old, 67 percent were African American, 28 percent lived below the federal poverty line. Like other American cities, New Orleans was a city of the many who were poor, the few who were rich, and the not-so-many in the middle who coped. Many of the latter had already fled to the suburbs and to surrounding small towns. After the hurricane more would follow, but now to distant places as well. New Orleans's "elite," still living in the city, was able to get out and, having places to go to, most did. To be sure, Katrina's outcomes had their antecedent causes, human causes. Not least of all, New Orleans was a tourist city with the low-paying service industries typical of tourist cities. Besides, the flooding was worse in the most vulnerable parts of town, particularly but not uniquely in the by-now notorious Ninth Ward. So, a not-so-latent racism—what those of us in the 1960s used to call "institutional racism"—exacerbated nature's destruction.

Looking back, Adam Nossiter of the *New York Times* would write,

> The struggle over housing in New Orleans raises the larger issue of how to reintegrate the most vulnerable residents after the hurricane; the ones most disrupted by the storm and still displaced 16 months later. And it has brought sharply into focus how much the New Orleans housing projects were places apart, vast islands of poverty in an already impoverished city. . . . "I think the romanticism that goes with the 'good old days of public housing' belies the harsh realities of crime and social malaise that had been created as a result of a concentration of low income folks," said Michael P. Kelly, who directed the troubled Housing Authority of New Orleans from 1995 to 2000 and now runs its counterpart in Washington, D.C. "Women who would put their babies in bathtubs at the sound of gunfire, that was a reality; coming home from your job and having to walk through young people participating in drug trades."[9]

The 100,000 waited. Over and over again, they heard rumors of rescue, but rumor was not fact. So, to the inherited cynicism of the black and the poor was added the failure of rescue and the anxieties of misinformation. The 100,000 were left in the dark in more ways than one. They were, above all, left to take care of themselves—but then there wasn't much new about that. Press, TV, and radio did great service in alerting the rest of the country, but with power out, broadcasts could hardly reach the 100,000. For five long days and more, they waited . . . in the Superdome with more than 20,000, in the Convention Center with as many, on the Highway I-10 overpasses where thousands more waited for evacuation after being rescued by boat and helicopter from rooftops and porches or pulled from the water. There were indeed a few buses commandeered unofficially by volunteers or sent from nearby cities and towns. The city's hundreds of school buses, however, were out of play. They had been parked for "safety" in a low-lying area and were inaccessible even if the order to use them had come. It did not. Many of the buses that finally did arrive were directed to places where the refugees were not or else they were held back to await official instructions. But, that also did not come. A few of the 455 buses ordered by FEMA started to arrive by Thursday, September 1st. In fact, however, it seemed to those left behind as if there were no buses!

> The governor of Louisiana was "blistering mad." It was the third night after Hurricane *Katrina* drowned New Orleans, and Gov. Kathleen Babineaux Blanco needed buses to rescue thousands of people from the fetid Superdome and convention center. But only a fraction of the 500 vehicles promised by federal authorities had arrived. Ms. Blanco burst into the state's emergency center in Baton Rouge. "Does anybody in this building know anything about buses?" she recalled crying out.[10]

FOOLS, VILLAINS, AND HEROES

Every catastrophe has its fools, and Katrina was no exception. As usual, there were those who boasted they would "ride-out" the storm only to find too late that this was a storm that did not suffer fools lightly. Others sought shelter in high-rise luxury hotels safely above the water only to find windows blown out, floors covered with broken glass, rooms flooded, generators running short of fuel, and water and food vanishing. Still others stayed home, trading the understandable and illusory security of the familiar for the actual insecurity of Katrina's chaos. Soon enough, they found themselves trying to move upward above the flood, although there wasn't much of an upward to move to in Ninth Ward's one-story housing. Desperately they waited to be saved before the surge engulfed their homes. Too often and for too many, help didn't arrive.

And then there was shelter. Officially, that was the Superdome, the "shelter of last resort." In his superb telling of Katrina's six days, Douglas Brinkley described it.

> The Superdome symbolized New Orleans as a big league city, the site of a 1987 visit from Pope John Paul II, the 1988 Republican National Convention, six Super Bowl games, and two NCAA Final Four basketball tournaments. Most famously, every January, the Sugar Bowl . . . was played there. Courtesy of *Katrina*, the Superdome's image changed overnight. *USA Today*, for instance, deemed it, "the epicenter of human misery." . . . People for the most part were taking care of their own," [NBC] newsman Brian Williams recalled. "But it was stifling hot inside. Some people were glad there was a hole in the roof because the rain cooled them off. Rumors of gangs were everywhere . . . The humidity was unbearable." . . . Senior citizens with respiratory problems couldn't take it. . . . According to Louisiana National Guard Colonel Thomas Beron. . . . "Don't get me wrong, bad things happened, but I didn't see any killing and raping and cutting throats or anything. . . . Ninety-nine percent of the people in the Dome were very well behaved."[11]

The Superdome was meant to shield people briefly until the hurricane's winds died down and the streets were safe to use. It became week-long living quarters for nearly 20,000 people, most of them African American. Rumor was everywhere and communication nowhere. Food and water were running out although there were enough military-style emergency rations to prevent starvation. Medical care was minimal. Stories of rape and murder spread fear in a crowded setting already fearful enough. However, as Colonel Beron of the National Guard tells us, the stories were untrue and the several hundred Louisiana National Guard troops assigned did manage to keep things somewhat orderly.

Soon enough, latecomers, seeing people turned away from the already overcrowded Superdome, moved on to the nearby Convention Center. Eventually there would be another 20,000 crowded into it. Unplanned for use as a shelter, nothing had been prepared . . . no food or water, no National Guard to keep order, no police, and "endless rooms running with open sewage" as Brinkley described it. Unlike the Superdome, violence and crime were real, not rumor. Gangs, as gangs will, established their turfs, defending them with threats and firearms. Not a few of the gangs, in an echo of medieval chivalry perhaps, protected the helpless—the women, the children, and the old.

Katrina had its heroes, too. The Louisiana Fish and Wildlife Department and the U.S. Coast Guard, the only government agencies that had boats available, saved thousands trapped in flooded neighborhoods. Coast Guard helicopters hoisted hundreds of frightened people from rooftops and attics. Nearly invisible was the city's mayor, who did not go to the Emergency

Operations Center. Instead, he remained in the Hyatt Hotel except for occasional and anonymous visits to the Superdome. There were the usual official meetings and conference calls and even a "summit" meeting on Air Force One. But often it seemed that these only delayed matters, using typical bureaucratic excuses. As meetings will: they offered the illusion of action where little or no action was taken.

> On Wednesday, August 31st, the President did a "fly-over" to view the devastation, not appearing on the ground in New Orleans until Friday, September 2nd, the fifth day after *Katrina* hit the Gulf coast. The military, bound by the *Posse Comitatus Act of 1878* was forbidden to engage in law enforcement and remained apart until, by Presidential order, army and marine units appeared on Saturday nearly a week after *Katrina* had struck. The police, many of whom, like other victims, had seen their homes destroyed, were almost invisible except for the very few who did not run away and who continued to "protect and serve" despite personal loss. The Louisiana National Guard weakened by duty in Iraq and in any case unprepared for such a catastrophe could provide only limited help. Two engineering battalions did make it to the Convention Center, they were specialists in clearing debris and not in disaster relief, so they isolated themselves and after less than 24 hours left. Ordinary citizens, one by one, rescued where and when they could, some had boats, others because of their familiarity with the city helping to find ways of getting to high ground. Over all, chaos and anarchy ruled.[12]

FEMA AND THE WAL-MART EXPRESS

The villain of the piece was FEMA [Federal Emergency Management Agency] and its Director, Michael Brown. Certainly, he was a likely scapegoat and as certainly, he earned the title. Trained as a lawyer, Brown was a political appointee with excellent Republican and conservative credentials, a pleasant manner, and little if any experience with disaster management. Appointed second in command at FEMA—he had also worked as a staff attorney there—he was named to the top post when Joseph Albaugh, another political appointee, left the job. Brown's earlier performance—a series of hurricanes in Florida in 2004—was adequate or at least the emergencies there were manageable. But that was Florida, a different geography, a different history of preparedness, a different number of refugees (20,000 and not 500,000), and not least of all a different governor and a different politics. After all, "04" was an election year, Florida was in play, and federal resources were quickly and competently made available.

Brown was not alone. In response to 9/11, the Department of Homeland Security [DHS] had been established. Along with many other agencies, FEMA was absorbed into it. The chain of command now ran to Michael

Chertoff and not directly to the president, as in Jimmy Carter's original design. Chertoff, a former judge and now Secretary of DHS, seemed as indifferent to the evolving catastrophe as did his subordinates and as did the president in those first strategic days when wind and water were destroying much of New Orleans and turning nearly half a million people into displaced persons. For good and not-so-good reasons, DHS and its top leadership was focused on terrorism. Realistic certainly, it was also "sexy" and politically appealing to a nation still reacting to the Twin Towers. "Ordinary" cataclysms like Katrina had lower priorities.

To his credit and whatever his lack of competence, Brown, when he found Chertoff unresponsive, made efforts to draw presidential and congressional attention to the realities on the ground. He was unsuccessful. No doubt in self-defense, he testified in early 2006 to congressional select committees on the federal response to Katrina, saying,

> It's my belief that had there been a report come out from Marty Bahamonde [FEMA's representative on site] that said, yes, we've confirmed that a terrorist has blown up the 17th Street Canal Levee, then everybody would have jumped all over that and been trying to do everything they could; but because this was a natural disaster, that has become a stepchild in the Department of Homeland Security; so you now have these two systems operating—one which cares about terrorism, and FEMA and our state and local partners, who are trying to approach everything from all hazards. And so there's this disconnect that exists within the system that we've created because of DHS.

But if Katrina was for Homeland Security only "an incident of significance," it was much more for the American community and not least of all for its corporations. Leading the way was Wal-Mart. It opened its warehouses to first responders, provided food and drink to the Gulf Coast states using its own trucks, and reassured its workers about the security of their jobs while giving them cash advances to tide them over. Above all, it demonstrated the management, organization, and logistics so glaringly absent in the government efforts. Wal-Mart "stepped over or around the confused, floundering, and sluggish bodies of federal, state, and local government relief agencies and sprang into action."[13] It had a lot of company. Among other businesses, Coca-Cola organized its own relief effort out of its headquarters in Atlanta. American Airlines evacuated its own workers and then, as soon as the New Orleans airport was reopened on September 30, sent food and medicines and helped evacuate refugees. Money to support nongovernmental agencies flowed freely from individual citizens, the states, religious and other organizations, and businesses—a billion plus dollars all told. On the ground, there was heroism enough from Public Health Service personnel, a few police, media reporters, and assorted volunteers. Houston became as it were an extension of New Orleans, accepting tens of thousands of refugees as evacuation took hold. Communities everywhere and not just in the South made homes available.

Summing it up, in February 2006, the Select Bipartisan Committee appointed to investigate the preparation for and response to Katrina issued its report, *A Failure of Initiative*. Among its conclusions,

- Failure to evacuate people led to preventable death, suffering, and delays in relief
- Critical National Response Plan elements were executed "late, ineffectively, or not at all"
- DHS and states were unprepared to deal with a catastrophic event of this magnitude
- Communications failures impaired response efforts
- Command and control at all levels did not function adequately, delaying relief
- The military was a valuable asset, but lacked coordination
- The lack of communication with the public and the absence of effective law enforcement led to civil unrest and further delayed relief efforts
- The medical community lacked adequate communications capabilities and advanced planning and had difficulty coordinating with authorities for relief
- FEMA's ability to provide emergency shelter and temporary housing was overwhelmed by the magnitude of the disaster and long-standing agency weaknesses
- FEMA logistics and contracting systems were insufficient for the magnitude of Hurricane Katrina
- Contributions from charitable organizations were generous, but in some cases, unorganized.

The report notes that "failure of local, state, and federal governments to respond more effectively to *Katrina*—which had been predicted in theory for many years, and forecast with startling accuracy for five days—demonstrates that whatever improvements have been made to our capacity to respond to natural or man-made disasters, four and half years after 9/11, we were still not fully prepared."[14]

KATRINA CONTINUES

Every disaster has its aftermath, the people displaced, the struggle to rebuild, the costs that were unmet, the lessons learned or ignored. And every disaster is both familiar and *sui generis*. Of course, we've seen big storms and big floods before. No catastrophe is without its echoes in time. Yet,

Katrina was different and not just because of its size and range and casualties. It also revealed the effects of a time of terrorism with its priorities and perceptions.

Katrina did not end with its six days of wind and water, the evacuations, the makeshift repair of the levees, and the receding floodwaters. Government at all levels had failed to do its job. The slow pace of response months after the opening acts of the disaster had passed reveals an unwillingness or inability to change. The reconstruction of the government agencies responsible for dealing with catastrophe is scarcely visible. DHS continues its terrorist priorities. FEMA, with new leadership, is slowly in the process of reform. But, remaining within DHS, there is little optimism for substantive change. The Corps of Engineers is still under-funded. Environmental damage is unchecked and, given the sentiment for rebuilding New Orleans as it was despite a loss of half of its population, will probably remained unchecked. The mayor, popular as ever, was re-elected. And besides, Iraq and soon enough Afghanistan have replaced Katrina as the crisis of the moment.

Housing and jobs remain a problem for tens of thousands—the media were filled for a time with pictures of thousands of mobile homes parked in vast storage areas, undistributed to people in need of shelter. Occasionally, stories appear recalling Katrina. But, except for a flurry of articles on the occasion of its second anniversary or when new hurricanes like Hannah and Ike in '08 occur, the media have moved on. Funds designated for relief are painfully slow in reaching those who need them. Insurance companies at first denied adequate coverage on the grounds—bless the lawyers—that hurricane insurance provides for wind damage but not for flood damage. Only two years later and under massive public pressure did they re-examine that judgment—as if Katrina's wind and water could be considered apart from each other.

Anecdotes tell us of refugees making new lives elsewhere, although dependable statistical information is still not available. Even those who have returned to rebuild their homes and their city are discouraged and are turning away.

> After nearly a decade in the city of their dreams, Kasandra Larsen and her fiancé, Dylan Langlois, climbed into a rented moving truck on Marais Street last Sunday, pointed it toward New Hampshire, and said goodbye. . . . A year ago, Ms. Larsen, 36, and Mr. Langlois, 37, were . . . eager to rebuild and improve the city they adored. But now they have joined hundreds of the city's best and brightest who . . . have made the wrenching decision to leave. . . . Their reasons include high crime, high rents, soaring insurance premiums and what many call a lack of leadership, competence, money and progress. . . . For every household that . . . has given up, there is another on the verge. Tyrone Wilson, a successful real estate agent and consultant, said he and his wife, Trina, a lawyer . . . "We came back, we tried," he said. . . .

> Low-income New Orleanians—those who will need the most help from a cash-strapped city—are making their way back, despite a lack of affordable housing. . . . Reganer Stewart, 30, a hotel maid, said she had been living with her cousin and her cousin's mother and four children since November. . . . Houston, which Ms. Stewart had not liked when she evacuated there, was growing more attractive as her search for an apartment here grew longer. "Most likely, we going to leave," she said. . . .
>
> The decision to leave is especially difficult for natives, said Elliott Stonecipher, a demographic analyst in Shreveport, La. . . . "They just won't talk about it; they do not want to talk about it," Mr. Stonecipher said. "It's remarkable that they just don't want anybody to know that they gave in."[15]

Health care is barely recovered. Metropolitan New Orleans had twenty-two hospitals, nine of them in the city. Eight months after Katrina, only fifteen of them had reopened, with 2,000 beds available where 4,400 had been available before. A report in the *New England Journal of Medicine* notes,

> Common themes at all facilities include complications in patients with untreated chronic diseases, particularly hypertension, diabetes, and AIDS. "These people come in with extremely severe problems," notes Alfred Abaunza, chief medical officer of *West Jefferson Medical Center*. "Diabetics have been off their insulin for six months. They come to us in diabetic ketoacidosis."[16]

Two years after the storm, "Only one of the city's seven general hospitals was operating at its pre-hurricane level; two more were partially open, and four remained closed. The number of hospital beds in New Orleans has dropped by two-thirds. In the suburbs, half a dozen hospitals in adjacent Jefferson Parish are open—but are packed."[17] With housing and jobs gone, most patients, again the black, the poor, and the old, have neither insurance nor other resources. The lack of access to health care for some forty-seven million is already a national scandal. In New Orleans and the delta, Katrina enlarged its effects. Hospitals, with Medicaid constrained by a shortage of state funds and reduced federal support, must treat without payment. Nursing home beds, always in short supply, are even more limited with consequent reduction in chronic care.

In addition, "New Orleans is experiencing what appears to be a near epidemic of depression and post-traumatic stress disorder . . . the local mental health system has suffered a near total collapse, heaping a great deal of the work to be done with emotionally disturbed residents onto the Police Department."[18] Tulane and Louisiana State University lost their psychiatric units in the storm. Psychiatrists and trained psychiatric nurses and nurse's aids are in short supply. As of the winter of 2007 only one-third of the city's schools had reopened. The rest, it is promised, will reopen in the fall. In short the people and the institutions that build and sustain communities—homes, jobs, health care, schools, and governments—continue to suffer the effects of Katrina and will for years to come.

Yet, there is hope. Adam Nossiter of the *New York Times*, who followed the story of Katrina from the beginning, reported,

> All over the city, a giant slow-motion reconstruction project is taking place. It is unplanned, fragmentary and for the isolated individuals carrying it out, often overwhelming. Those with the fortitude to persevere—and only the hardiest even try—must battle the hopelessness brought on by a continuing sense of abandonment. The selection process has been Darwinian, with a combination of drive, tenacity, luck and savings seeing the neo-colonizers through. . . . A few thousand hammers and nails, of course, go only so far in a city that remains stricken nearly two years after the *Katrina* floodwaters. . . . Though neighborhoods are shells of what they were, they have not disappeared.[19]

And there is even some hope of effective help for other cities facing other Katrinas. For example, while far less destructive, Hurricane Gustav and Tropical Storm Ike in the fall of 2008 revealed that FEMA and the White House have learned to do a bit better if for no other reason than to avoid the political fallout of another Katrina. At the same time, the levees were deliberately rebuilt by the Corps of Engineers, but not strongly enough to withstand another Katrina. The money, they tell us, was not available. So we learn, but we do not really learn.

THE LOST COMMUNITY

But what has all of this have to do with bioethics? Returning to the Aristotelian necessity with which I began this chapter, healthy persons require healthy communities and healthy communities require healthy persons. Indeed, empirical studies verify this connection.[20] Where that connection is broken, health becomes an elusive ideal and pathology a social norm. With this in mind, let me touch explicitly on the issues embedded in the Katrina narrative, many of which will reappear as we look at other moments of disaster. The first and most basic is trust in public institutions and in each other. Already shaky—minorities typically have a cynical view of governments—the failures of Katrina and its aftermath have confirmed them in that cynicism. Even more telling, the middle class as we have seen is also moving from skepticism to that same cynicism. As David Brooks, a conservative *New York Times* columnist, put it,

> The first rule of the social fabric—that in times of crisis you protect the vulnerable—was trampled. Leaving the poor in New Orleans was the moral equivalent of leaving the injured on the battlefield. No wonder confidence in civic

institutions is plummeting. . . . It's already clear this will be known as the grueling decade, the Hobbesian decade. Americans have had to acknowledge dark realities that it is not in our nature to readily acknowledge: the thin veneer of civilization, the elemental violence in human nature, the lurking ferocity of the environment, the limitations on what we can plan and know, the cumbersome reactions of bureaucracies, the uncertain progress good makes over evil.[21]

Failure to perform is the root source of skepticism. Repeated false and empty promises move us toward cynicism. Nor is the situation helped by the fact, appearing over and over again in the Katrina story, that truthful and widely shared communication was minimal at best. Rumor took its place, and this only added to the natural anxiety and fear of those left behind. Judging these failures by bioethical values is hardly difficult. Respect for persons as in autonomy and informed consent cannot survive in such a climate. Without commitment to the dignity of persons, caregivers cannot do their work and disaster's victims cannot be effectively served. Those done-to and those doing-for are both disabled.

Closely tied to trust is competence. But, the story of Katrina is, by and large, a story of incompetence where a democracy needs it most—in its government, its policies, and it decision-makers. To be sure, we do not think of competence as a moral category. We think of it in more "objective" terms, as something rooted in knowledge and measured by performance. "Outcome" is biomedicine's term of art. As it turns out, however, this "objectivity" misleads, and consequently, the lessons of Katrina are not learned. Ethics becomes a luxury in the face of catastrophe. Judgment becomes only accusatory, and action is reduced to bloodless technique. Moral agency is thus disconnected from effectiveness. Again, Whitehead is helpful, "Duty arises from our potential control over the course of events. Where attainable knowledge could have changed the issue, ignorance has the guilt of vice."[22]

And then there is authority, another moral term in trust's moral lexicon. Were it not so deadly, the confusions of jurisdiction and the not-so-hidden political gamesmanship evident in Katrina would warrant a farce. Perhaps, in time, that farce will be written. Authority—more familiarly, leadership—is one of the great problems of ethics; that is, the search for legitimacy and, in our setting, the demands of democratic legitimacy. Failure here, the failure of authority to be accountable, to be authoritative in short, transforms chaotic events into chaos. Surely Katrina's experience of governmental failure and leadership abdication provides instance enough of this transformation.

Finally, there is history and metaphysics, strange intrusions into bioethics! Yet, race and class, New Orleans's demography, haunt Katrina and its aftermath. The sense of place and displacement that shaped evacuation, return, and unwilling displacement again ask for a philosophic, even spiritual, anthropology. And our offenses, the vanishing delta as symbol and as reality, beg for a critical naturalistic metaphysics. As it were, mental health was not only a clinical issue but also an existential one. The fracture of self, community, and nature, Katrina's deeper reality, has yet to find its therapy.

NOTES

1. "A City Beyond the Reach of Empathy," Richard Ford, *NYT*, 9/4/05.

2. Jonathan Moreno at the University of Virginia has raised similar questions about the narrowness that all too often afflicts what we call "biomedical ethics." In doing so, he calls us back to an earlier wisdom, i.e., Van Rensselaer Potter's "bioethics" and the effort "to achieve a more generous agenda . . . in Peter Whitehouse's recent concise formulation, the 'integration of biology and values . . . designed to guide human survival.'" "In the Wake of Katrina: Has 'Bioethics' Failed?" Jonathan D. Moreno, *AJOB*, Jan/Feb 2006.

3. The precipitating event for me was my participation in planning and helping to teach a pilot course on "Ethics and Preparedness in an Age of Terrorism," sponsored by the Center for Public Health Preparedness at the Arnold School of Public Health, University of South Carolina. After its demonstrated effectiveness, I was responsible for preparing a textbook for the course (available as a CD and distributed by the Center for Preparedness, School of Public Health, University of South Carolina, Columbia, SC).

4. For example, three years later, in September 2008, Hurricane Gustav struck near New Orleans. But the levees held; there was no panic, only one reported case of looting, and nearly two million people were successfully evacuated. Ultimately, Gustav missed the city. But compounding the situation was that waiting in the wings were Hurricane Hanna and Tropical Storm Ike. As National Public Radio reported (September 1, 2008),

> The brutal memories of Katrina which flooded nearly 80 percent of New Orleans and killed more than 1,600 along the Gulf Coast, led officials to insist that everyone in Gustav's path flee from the shore . . . President Bush, eager to show that the mistakes with Hurricane Katrina in 2005 would not be repeated, visited emergency response centers in Texas. . . . After Hurricane Katrina in 2005, more than 100,000 families were left homeless and ended up in travel trailers or mobile homes provided by the Federal Emergency Management Agency. Federal authorities say they won't use the trailers again unless absolutely necessary because of concerns about high formaldehyde fumes inside.

5. For example, the 2004 tsunami struck eleven countries in South Asia, resulted in some 150,000 deaths, tens of thousands missing, hundreds of thousands of survivors without homes or livelihood.

6. Published a few days before Katrina struck, the article was written months before. "Drowning New Orleans," Mark Fischetti, *Scientific American*, 8/31/05. (A major hurricane could swamp New Orleans under twenty feet of water, killing thousands. Human activities along the Mississippi River have dramatically increased the risk, and now only massive reengineering of southeastern Louisiana can save the city.)

7. Asked to explain its failure to protect New Orleans from flooding, the Army Corps of Engineers produced an answer yesterday [July 10, 2007]: "Bit by bit over some 50 years, the corps made a series of decisions based largely on dollars, politics and scheduling . . the system originally envisioned when Congress authorized the construction of the series of levees, floodwalls and storm gates was very different from what the Corps ultimately delivered. Again and again. Corps officials decided to push forward with the plan they had rather than change course, incur greater costs and further delays and risk the wrath of Congress, which would have had to authorize the additional financing. When they did change course—often under pressure from federal and local officials—the changes appear to have increased the risk to the city."

"Engineers Faulted on Hurricane System," John Schwartz, *NYT*, 7/11/07.

8. National Weather Service, New Orleans, August 28, 2005.

9. "In New Orleans, Some Hope of Taking Back the Projects," Adam Nossiter, *NYT*, 12/26/06.

10. "Breakdowns Marked Path from Hurricane to Anarchy," Eric Lipton, Christopher Drew, Scott Shane, and David Rohde, *NYT*, 9/11/05.

11. *The Great Deluge*, Douglas Brinkley, Harper Collins, 2006, pp. 192–93.

12. For a striking and disheartening description of what happened at the Convention Center, see Brinkley, pp. 273–80.

13. "Government Can Take Lesson from Wal-Mart," Bill Steigerwald, *Pittsburgh Tribune-Review*, 10/14/05.

14. "Bipartisan Report Finds Failures at All Levels of Government in Hurricane Response," *Biosecurity Briefing* [University of Pittsburgh], 2/17/06. (*A Failure of Initiative: The Final Report of the Select Bipartisan Committee to Investigate the Preparation for and Response to Hurricane Katrina*, 2/15/06.)

15. "In Setback for New Orleans, Fed-Up Residents Give Up," Shaila Dewan, *NYT*, 2/16/07.

16. "After the Storm—Health Care Infrastructure in Post-Katrina New Orleans," Ruth E. Berggren and Tyler J. Curiel, *NEJM*, Vol 354, 15, 04/13/06, 1549–52.

17. "Recovery in New Orleans Is Slowed by Closed Hospitals," Leslie Eaton, *NYT*, 7/24/07.

18. "A Legacy of the Storm: Depression and Suicide," Susan Saulny, *NYT*, 6/23/06.

19. "Patchwork City, Largely Alone, Pioneers Reclaim New Orleans," Adam Nossiter, *NYT*, 7/2/07.

20. "Health Effects of Housing Improvement: Systematic Review of Intervention Studies," Hilary Thomson, Higher Scientific Officer, Mark Petticrew, Associate Director, David Morrison, Specialist Registrar in Public Health Medicine, *BMJ*, 323 (7306)2001, 187, 07/28/01.

21. "The Bursting Point," David Brooks, *NYT*, 9/4/05.

22. *The Aims of Education*, Alfred North Whitehead, New American Library, MacMillan, 1949, p. 26.

5

The Case of Dr. Pou

Warrant of Arrest

To: Any Law Enforcement Officer:

Affidavit having been made by Special Agent Virginia B. Rider of the Louisiana Department of Justice, Criminal Division, Medicaid Fraud Control Unit, that on or about September 1, 2005, the offender, Anna M. Pou, 928 Louisiana Avenue, New Orleans, LA 70115, did commit the crime of Principal to Second Degree Murder, four counts, by intentionally killing four patients at Memorial Medical Center, New Orleans, LA, by administering or causing to be administered lethal doses of morphine sulphate (morphine) and midazolam (Versed), as defined in Louisiana Revised Statute 14:24 and 14:30.1.

You are, therefore, commanded forthwith to arrest the said offender and take her forthwith to be booked and charged in accordance with the law.

Dated in New Orleans, Louisiana, this 17th day of July, 2006.

Every catastrophe has its victims. Typically, we hardly know their names. Instead, they serve as counters in measuring disaster's magnitude. Scarcely thinking it strange, our vocabulary becomes arithmetical—so many dead, so many injured, so many saved, so many houses destroyed, so many trees downed, so many dollars lost, and so on. Of course, there are lists of names for the record, but rarely do they touch us unless we have a personal connection. After a while, the lists blur, becoming no more communicative than the numbers. It is the rare exception, like the Vietnam Memorial or the ceremonial reading of the names of the dead on 9/11's anniversary, that converts lists into mourning and remembrance. Yet, every victim has a name and a biography. So too with Katrina and, save for its public heroes, fools, and villains, so too with its nameless ones.[1] Hence, this chapter.

There is comfort in lists, the protection of anonymity and the safety of numbers. Lacking personal identity, we can easily put victims aside. The suffering measured by lists is all too easily dulled by memory turned generic. Katrina also imports a certain shame—too many failed and too many waited for help that never came—a nation's shame for an America whose illusion is "can do" and whose myth is "superpower." Apt echo to Katrina, I hear again Shelley's *Ozymandias,*

I met a traveler from an antique land
Who said:—Two vast and trunkless legs of stone
Stand in the desert. Near them on the sand,
Half sunk, a shatter'd visage lies, whose frown
And wrinkled lip and sneer of cold command
Tell that its sculptor well those passions read
Which yet survive, stamp'd on these lifeless things,
The hand that mock'd them and the heart that fed.
And on the pedestal these words appear:
"My name is Ozymandias, king of kings:
Look on my works, ye mighty, and despair!"
Nothing beside remains: round the decay
Of that colossal wreck, boundless and bare,
The lone and level sands stretch far away.

To disaster's event is joined Katrina's aftertime. It is not over when it's over, and the "fat lady" hasn't sung her last song yet. Lists become insufficient, unsatisfying. Proper names return to consciousness. Meanwhile, the stars of the piece, so to speak—Negin and Blanco and Brown, and yes, Chertoff and Bush—beg for the ministrations of Jonathan Swift or Gilbert and Sullivan. Of course, farce is not enough, although ridicule for the politician is surely no trivial matter. In the aftertime, others, more ambiguously identified, enter the scene. Thus, the setting for Dr. Anna Pou and the nurses, Lori Budo and Cheri Landry, for Attorney General Charles Foti and, silently present, for the four dead patients on the seventh floor.

Even now, three years later as I write, it is not entirely clear how this drama will finally play out. The affidavit was published, the arrest was made, but the District Attorney hesitated. A grand jury was finally convened in March of 2007. Landry and Budo were granted immunity so that they could testify without risking self-incrimination. No surprise, Dr. Pou stood alone.

Four months later, on July 24, the grand jury announced that it would not indict. Dr. Pou was free at last of the threat of imprisonment. Landry and Budo returned to that anonymity our habits accord to nurses, as if they were only minor players.

But the story is still not over. Three of the families have sued Dr. Pou in civil court. Dr. Pou has sued the state of Louisiana in order to recover her legal costs. Five outside forensic experts have examined the corpses. None of the experts, apparently, was called to testify. In media interviews, they reported that as many as nine patients had been killed with overdoses of drugs, so homicide should not be ruled out. In the beginning, the Attorney General had called the cause of death a "lethal cocktail." The District Attorney, however, refused to comment on the grounds that grand jury proceedings were confidential.

Other experts, not the state's, argue that, "blood levels of morphine are greatly increased in patients who have been dead for many days."[2] They add that morphine dosages are adjusted to a patient's needs and history, information only partly available to Dr. Pou in the chaos of Katrina. For example, Dr. Steven Miles, professor of Medicine at the University of Minnesota and an expert on the care of dying patients, said, "The selection of drugs looks to me to be more typical of the drugs selected for providing palliative care rather than killing patients." Earlier, R. Alta Charo, professor of Law and Bioethics at the University of Wisconsin, had said, "The real dilemma here is in getting at the very precise facts of the case. I can say that, as a general matter, if you have a patient who is in distress and who needs pain relief and if the only level of painkillers that will relieve the pain also poses a high risk of death then it is permissible to give the pain relievers, provided the patient has consented to the risk of death. Even if the patient can no longer give consent . . . it is still ethical for doctors to treat the pain if they believe it is what the patient would want."[3]

HOSPITALS

As the levees failed, each New Orleans hospital faced the problem of how to care for its patients. Each tried to evacuate them and its staff to safety. Each also faced anxious families, grown more anxious as the doors were shut and communication failed. Each had to turn away hundreds of others seeking shelter in hospitals that were seen as islands of safety. Each hospital faced staff members worried about their families and their own survival. As the hours went by, each hospital found itself, having barred its doors, less and less able to do what it was committed to do, to provide care and comfort to desperate people.

Of the nine New Orleans hospitals, some did better than others, were better prepared than others, or were just luckier than others. Sadly, there was no coordinated plan in place—typically the responsibility of governments in an emergency—for assessing needs and numbers, for securing necessary resources, and for organizing evacuation. In short, each hospital was pretty much on its own, forced to make do with what it had or with what happened to come its way. A volunteer physician at Tulane Hospital wrote,

> Katrina's floodwaters crippled emergency power generators, transforming hospitals into dark, fetid, dangerous shells. Extremely high indoor temperatures killed some people. We were under tremendous strain: in addition to the dire medical circumstances of many of our patients, we confronted uncertainty about our own evacuation, exacerbated by the tensions of threatened violence by snipers and frazzled soldiers and guards. I saw some competent professionals reduced to utter incoherence and uselessness as the crisis unfolded. I saw others perform heroic deeds that surprised me.[4]

Memorial Medical Center, a for-profit hospital owned by Tenet Corporation, was in no better and no worse shape than the other eight. Like them it was a refuge that couldn't offer refuge. Like them, the power had failed and the batteries that were to provide for emergencies were running low. The technology on which so much of medicine depends these days was rapidly becoming unavailable. Air conditioning was unavailable, too. Temperatures rose above one hundred degrees and stayed there with minor relief at night for five long days. Sewers, dependent on pumps also powered by electricity, backed up. The dead, with no place else to go, were put in the chapel to wait. Their decaying corpses added to the smells of sewage and the effects on hundreds of human bodies of day after day of unbearable heat and the lack of bath water. Medicines, food, and drinking water were running low. It was like practicing medicine "as if in a third world country," said one physician. Surrounded by flood and with resources vanishing, Memorial's staff tried to care for its 260 patients. At last, evacuation began on Wednesday, three days after Katrina struck and the levees broke. Forty-five bodies were left behind, to be removed later.

Memorial had another problem. It was not in control of all of its units. LifeCare Hospitals leased space from it in order to serve geriatric patients.[5] Having evacuated its hospital in Chalmette, a nearby delta town, before the storm, it had sent its patients to Memorial. With its own staff and administration, LifeCare made its decisions on how to deal with the situation. To be sure, it tried to coordinate its plans with Memorial, but in the chaos of Katrina and given the special needs of geriatric patients, that didn't work out very well.

LifeCare's most vulnerable patients were in a unit on Memorial's seventh floor. Sick and elderly, with limited or no mobility, evacuation by raft and boat wouldn't work for them. Helicopters might have taken them to shelters out of the city. But, helicopters arrived haphazardly, unpredictably, if at all. Even when they did, they needed to land on the roof of the hospital's garage building. But, there was no direct access to the roof and the elevators weren't working. The seventh-floor patients would have had to be carried down the stairs to the second floor of the hospital building, then through a three-by-three foot hole that had been broken open in the wall between the hospital and the garage, and finally up the ramps to the garage roof. For the few caregivers who volunteered to stay behind, the task would have been impossible and the results for many of the patients deadly. In fact, twenty-four of the fifty-five patients in the LifeCare units died. Four of them, however, were rumored to be victims of euthanasia. The other twenty were presumed to be victims of their fragility in conditions where fragility was fatal.

THE SEVENTH FLOOR

On Saturday, August 27, Anna Pou, a surgeon whose specialty was endocrinology, arrived at Memorial to see her patients. On call for that weekend, she remained at the hospital until Thursday, September 1, after all patients still alive—some forty-five Memorial patients had died—and staff had been evacuated. By that time, she, Cheri Landry, and Lori Budo were the only ones left on the seventh floor. LifeCare personnel were gone. They had been told to leave by their administrators who had, according to the affidavit, been informed by Dr. Pou that she and the two nurses would take care of the remaining patients. Perhaps there was miscommunication. Perhaps the LifeCare administrators were protecting themselves and their institution from the lawsuits that would no doubt follow. We simply do not know. But, unless some monstrous intention motivated Dr. Pou, it seems more than likely that a "duty to treat" kept her and Budo and Landry at work while others left.[6]

Dr. Pou is a native of New Orleans. Her father and uncle are both physicians. She trained at Louisiana State, had residencies and fellowships in Memphis, Pittsburgh, and Indiana. After five years of teaching at the University of Texas Medical School in Galveston, she returned to practice in New Orleans in 2004. A teacher and an author of a number of research articles—her resumé runs to twenty-one pages—she was known as a patient advocate, a dedicated physician, and a dependable colleague. Apart from their names, titles, and degrees, the nurses are nearly anonymous. Indeed, except ironically for the "Order of Arrest," most of the reports of the case simply refer to them as "Dr. Pou and two nurses."

The four patients who are the alleged murder victims would in all probability not have survived the rigors of evacuation even if helicopters had been accessible. Of the four, one was sixty-one, paralyzed, and weighed 380 pounds; another was sixty-six; another was eighty-nine and had gangrene in both legs and suffered from dementia; and another was ninety and had bronchitis but was otherwise stable. As Dr. Pou reported, she and the nurses decided to provide palliative (comfort) care as the only medically indicated treatment available to them; that is, morphine for relief of pain and Versed (midazolam) for relief of anxiety. Ultimately, Pou, Budo, and Landry did not leave the hospital until all patients were either evacuated or dead.

ACCUSATION

We will probably never know exactly what happened on the seventh floor during the Wednesday and Thursday evacuation. The reports tell a mixed and contradictory tale. For example, the state's forensic experts refer to nine patients, the affidavit to four. The witness testimony cited in the affidavit stops just short of accusation. Some reports describe the four patients as DNR (Do Not Resuscitate). Some describe them as "chronic," while others describe them as "acute." No one, however, denies three facts: Pou, Budo, and Landry volunteered to stay while everyone else left; the patients were in a rapidly deteriorating condition; and they did receive injections of morphine and Versed. Beyond that we have rumor, allegation, and guesswork. National Public Radio reported,

> Soon after Hurricane Katrina struck, the first unconfirmed reports surfaced of "mercy killings" . . . at New Orleans hospitals. For months, the Louisiana attorney general has been investigating these charges. That investigation has centered on the actions of doctors and nurses at the city's Memorial Medical Center. There, on the seventh floor conditions were deteriorating rapidly, evacuations were sporadic and security was compromised. Staff agonized whether to attempt to transport critically ill patients who might not survive the arduous evacuation. It appears another choice was considered: whether to end the lives of those who could not be moved. In the court documents . . . none of four key witnesses say they knew who made the decision to administer lethal doses of painkillers to the patients. But all four heard discussions that a decision had been made to end patients' lives.[7]

In the *New England Journal of Medicine*, Tyler Curiel wrote,

> "Patients were complaining some," reported one of Lambert's colleagues, "but we never considered euthanasia." . . . Lambert [Colleen Lambert, a nurse at Memorial's transplant unit] . . . acknowledged that she "did hear rumors" 3 days after Katrina that "they're talking about euthanizing patients," but that discussion apparently centered only on patients in the LifeCare facility. She said she was not entirely surprised, given what she had heard about conditions there.[8]

Frank Dawkins, an attorney, summed it up,

> According to the affidavit for the arrest warrants, Pou allegedly told T. M., nurse executive and director of education of LifeCare Hospitals . . . on the morning of September 1, 2005, that "a decision had been made to administer lethal doses" to the four critically-ill patients. Allegedly, T. M. asked Pou "Lethal doses of what?" T. M. did not recall Pou's exact response, but "believes" she said "morphine and Ativan (lorazepam)." Additionally, the affidavit alleges that S. H., the pharmacy director for LifeCare Hospitals, and D. R., assistant administrator for Lifecare Hospitals, also were informed that morning by Dr. Pou "that a decision had been made to administer lethal doses to the LifeCare patients remaining on the seventh floor."[9]

It is not surprising that the families of three of the patients who were supposed to have been euthanized had expressed their anger publicly. "She didn't act like a 90-year-old," J. C. said of her mother. "She was all there. She knew where she was. She knew who she was." The daughter of another patient said that "her mother . . . had been very sick, with gangrene in both legs and dementia, but that she had been stable two days before Katrina hit. 89 [years old], [she] had been scheduled to have her legs amputated August 29, the day the hurricane hit." The widow of the third patient, sixty-one-years old . . . "declined to comment. . . . [He] was 380 pounds and paralyzed, appeared 'conscious, awake and alert' before he was sedated, according to the arrest affidavit."[10]

Charles Foti, the Louisiana Attorney General, a long-time advocate for the rights of the elderly, noted that he was required by law to conduct an investigation if bona fide complaints were made.[11] Since family members did complain and since both LifeCare and Memorial "self-reported" their concerns, it would seem that he had little choice but to investigate. Over a ten-month period, Foti's investigation is said to have heard one hundred witnesses. Of that number, however, only four, the LifeCare administrators, are cited extensively in the affidavit. In a news conference, he would not comment on a motive for the killings. He did, however, say, "This is not euthanasia, this is plain and simple homicide."[12]

Two months later, on September 24th, Dr. Pou appeared on CBS's *60 Minutes*. The Associated Press quoted her,

> "I want everyone to know that I am not a murderer. That we are not murderers," says Dr. Anna Pou, who, along with nurses Cheri Landry and Lori Budo, was arrested and booked on second-degree murder charges July 17. "I do not believe in euthanasia," said Pou. "I have spent my entire life taking care of patients. I have no history of doing anything other than good for my patients. . . . Why would I suddenly start murdering people?" Her goal was to "ensure they do not suffer in pain." Pou acknowledges the drugs could have caused harm, but stresses: "Anytime you provide pain medicine to anybody, there is a risk. But as I said, my role is to help them through the pain."[13]

In the same interview, Attorney General Foti stated, "When you use both of them (morphine and Versed) together it becomes a lethal cocktail and guarantees they're going to die." A few days later, in rebuttal, the Louisiana State Medical Society issued a statement in support of Dr. Pou. It read in part,

> The Louisiana State Medical Society (LSMS) is confident that Dr. Pou performed courageously under the most challenging and horrific conditions and made decisions in the best interest of her patients. . . . Her long and distinguished career as a talented surgeon and dedicated educator should not be tarnished as a result of these accusations. Dr. Pou is entitled to the presumption of innocence. . . . The Louisiana State Medical Society will continue to support Dr. Pou as she has always supported her patients.[14]

The American Medical Association urged that there not be a rush to judgment. Many of Dr. Pou's colleagues expressed public confidence in both her abilities and her professional and personal ethics. Letters in the local press, many from Dr. Pou's patients, were unanimous in their support.

THE MORAL OF THE STORY IS . . .

Pou, Budo, and Landry were faced with a choice of evils, at best. In the conditions they faced, honest and complete information was urgently needed. But information—about rescue, about resources—didn't come. The little that did get through was incomplete, and rumor replaced fact. Yet, they had to decide. Doing nothing would, in itself, have been a decision. On the seventh floor, it would have been the equivalent of abandonment, a morally dubious decision.

And for the rest of us, how shall we judge? The evidence is confusing. Memories are colored by time and desire. For some, they grow vague as time passes. For others, paradoxically, memory claims a clarity that in all probability was absent closer to the event. Personal history, perspective, position, and self-interest shape recollection and shape what and how we receive it. Witnesses, in short, are notoriously unreliable and even more so with the passage of time.

Sorting out some, but only some, of the issues that Katrina's chaos and Pou's choices present is, of necessity, an exercise in imperfection. If a failure of trust is the message of Katrina, then a failure of responsibility is the message of Memorial and LifeCare.

A look at actual and potential consequences of the choices before Pou, Budo, and Landry opens up another moral question. Difficult enough under "normal" conditions, can we rely on our moral habits and "standard of care" when chaos shapes the scene? Moral language is not self-defining even under ordinary conditions. For example, what does "harm" mean when, following Hippocrates, we agree, "first do no harm"? Moral habit becomes even more problematic under emergency conditions. Triage sacrifices some in order to save others. And it becomes almost unintelligible when emergency becomes catastrophe. Epistemic convenience, the possibility of dealing with moral issues neatly, vanishes. We are all too easily trapped by the law into a false clarity.

"JUST THE FACTS, MA'AM."

Facts neither select themselves nor speak for themselves. While I suspect the presence of political motives—Attorney General Foti was up for re-election—I have sympathy for him as well. He was after all obligated by his office to find out what happened on the seventh floor. Like you and me, he probably said to himself something like, four people are dead under questionable circumstances and that ought not go unnoticed just because other deaths were caused by wind and flood. Something separates what happened on the seventh floor from these other deaths. In short, who or what was responsible? But the question does not allow an easy answer. Incompetence, as we have seen, certainly played a role in the Katrina event. But, incompetence ordinarily lacks intention and will, and it is, these that signal moral agency.[15] Negin, Blanco, and Brown, however, held public office. They were required by their roles to have known better and done better. Incompetence thus shifts to irresponsibility. Indeed they could not avoid knowing better given the predictions that had been made many times over the years. But, they were not alone. Decisions made long ago—and still being made today after Katrina—about budgets and levees and housing introduce an entire city to culpability—engineers and politicos and ordinary citizens, too.

Avoidable ignorance surely contributed, indirectly at least, to all the deaths of Katrina and not just to the four deaths on the seventh floor. This raises a related but separate set of moral considerations, the problem of the complicit community.[16] But, whatever others may have done or failed to do, we still need to assess personal responsibility where we can. Thus, from a moral point of view, we are not excused from exploring the complaint against Pou, Budo, and Landry. At the same time, I detect a resort to scapegoats. I cannot help but remark that no public officials or hospital administrators faced a charge of murder or even of contributory negligence. At worst, except for Negin who was re-elected, they may have lost their jobs.

Responsibility is an inclusive category. Moral agency, much narrower, stands or falls on causality and intention. Did these four patients have to die and did the three caregivers willfully and deliberately act to make them die? The Attorney General says yes, The DA and Grand Jury say no. There will be no indictment and no criminal trial. But ethics asks for more nuanced consideration, i.e., about the culpability of ignorance, about the politics of negligence and about the psychology of denial, and about the seventh floor in a catastrophic setting.

Pou, Budo, and Landry could not avoid decision on September 1st. The simple fact that they volunteered to stay behind when just about all others had left verifies that conclusion. Perhaps they made wrong decisions, even mistaken ones. But the information on which their decisions were based was surely flawed. No remedy for that was available to them. So moral fault without the possibility of adequate knowledge is a dubious conclusion.

Just about all references in the public arena focus on the patients as victims. Unmentioned is the vulnerability of the caregivers, as if they were somehow immune to chaos. Yet, they too were in danger. They too must have experienced anxiety personally and frustration professionally, i.e., the need to treat without the tools of treatment. They too must have felt isolated and abandoned. The myth of the godlike and objective professional may work well enough under normal conditions. It is naïve, however, to assume that chaos had no effect on Pou, Budo, and Landry.

Although rescue did arrive a day later, Pou, Budo, and Landry could not have known that. They had concluded from the information they did have that it would not come in time and that, in any event, the four patients were moving rapidly beyond rescue. If not in "terminal" condition clinically, they were surely in terminal condition existentially. The issue for the three caregivers thus became, what would ease their patient's dying and how would these patients die—peaceably or painfully in a situation of unbearable heat and humidity, dehydration, and starvation. The caregivers surely had guidance on how we deal with withholding or withdrawing treatment, with comfort care and with "terminal sedation."[17] These choices are difficult enough under "normal" conditions. Chaos confounds the situation.

The options on the seventh floor had reduced to doing nothing, giving comfort care but only as long as medication was available, or ultimately euthanasia. Dr. Pou clearly opted against abandonment. The medical record does not unequivocally support a choice for euthanasia. She claims she chose comfort care and except for self-interested testimony, rumor, and hearsay, the record does not dispute her. In an effort to secure consent for treatment, we know that Dr. Pou had tried to have a LifeCare nurse discuss the situation with one of the patients who was lucid and "decisional," as the jargon goes. We know too, that the nurse refused. We do not know if, later on, the patients were asked for their consent to one or another of these options. We can speculate, based on the record that, by then, Dr. Pou had concluded that at least three of these patients if not all four were no longer coherent enough to give informed consent.

If this is a fair way of thinking about the case—and I think it is—then we might look to how we make choices when facing predictions about the end of life. Certainly, we rely on colleagues and families. Where a patient is unable to make decisions, we seek surrogate decision-makers. In short, we neither judge nor decide nor act alone. But on the seventh floor all but the three caregivers and the patients were gone. It and they were isolated. Pou, Budo, and Landry didn't have the option of consultation or the luxury of time.

We grant permission to act according to our estimate of a patient's best interests a life-threatening emergency when a patient is incapable of informed choice. Under such circumstance, informed consent is presumed. If Dr. Pou's comments are believed, "comfort care"—sedation—became her only legitimate professional choice. But that did not end her difficulties. Determining appropriate level of sedation is a subtle art. Yet none of the three caregivers had a history with these patients. They had to rely on guesswork and experience. Too much or too little sedation would not have been surprising. The affidavit suggests this interpretation when it notes,

> [At a meeting on Thursday morning] Susan Mulderick, Incident Commander for Memorial Medical Center, advised participants she was aware LifeCare had nine critical patients [?] on the seventh floor. Ms. Mulderick stated she did not expect these patients would be evacuated with the rest of the hospital. . . . Later that morning, S.H., K.J. and D.R. [all LifeCare administrators] spoke with Ms. Mulderick again. Ms. Mulderick advised that some decisions had been made regarding the LifeCare patients and they should speak with Dr. Pou . . . Dr. Pou informed S.H. and D.R. that a decision had been made to administer lethal doses to the LifeCare patients remaining on the seventh floor. D.R. brought up the fact that patient E.E. was alert and oriented. Dr. Pou asked if someone from LifeCare could talk with E.E. or sedate him. Initially someone mentioned that A.G., a LifeCare RN, had a close relationship with E.E., but A.G. refused to participate in sedating E.E. At that point, D.R. decided that no LifeCare staff should be involved.[18]

However we ultimately assess the acts and intentions of Pou, Budo, and Landry, several things emerge clearly. All three were volunteers, and all three were at risk. Memorial patients and staff had been evacuated. The other LifeCare patients and all of LifeCare's staff had been evacuated. The affidavit does not tell us how many other caregivers were left in the hospital—in the various available descriptions, reference is only to "a few." In any event, we do know that Pou and the two nurses were the only ones remaining to tend to the LifeCare patients on the seventh floor. As the state Medical Society put it, Dr. Pou "performed courageously under the most challenging and horrific conditions and made decisions in the best interest of her patients." The same should be said of nurses Budo and Landry.

It is difficult to avoid the conclusion that LifeCare, in ordering its staff to leave, had in effect deserted its seventh-floor patients. To be sure, they had provided for a transfer of responsibility. But it was surely an imperfect transfer. LifeCare staff had turned over to strangers patients in extreme condition and in a terrifying situation. Its administrators had passed responsibility to a physician and two nurses who were not specialized in geriatric care and who did not know these patients. As an attorney remarked to me, perhaps unfairly, after reviewing the affidavit, LifeCare seemed more concerned with protecting itself—against criticism and against civil suit—than it was with protecting its patients.

It is tempting to shift responsibility from Pou, Budo, and Landry to LifeCare and its administrators. But the administrators might well have been caught between their professional and their institutional obligations. Before playing the "blame game," it is worth reminding ourselves of the problem of causality and culpability. Thus, a comment by a physician,

> I look at virtually all the deaths of Katrina as a consequence of system problem. . . . I can see that the deaths, probably the majority were related directly to this system failure. . . . If this assumption is correct, then if one was to find behavior that lead to these deaths of Katrina one would have to consider all the levels of the system. Surely, considering the ethical principle of justice, if punishment is to be meted out to those who contributed to the deaths, certainly other individuals at all levels of the system and their actions should also be investigated beyond the doctor and two nurses. Most of those who died, I can assume, did not die a natural death but died because the system didn't work.[19]

Perhaps then there were no villains, or perhaps there were too many. If so, agency takes on extended meaning and is perhaps stretched so far as to become unintelligible. To avoid the problem, we might choose to adopt the notion of a "chain of command" to the ethics of chaos. At the top, separated from the frantic action on the ground, leadership carries the burden of judgment and decision; its intentions become everyone's intentions. But in practice hierarchy is truncated for political or other reasons, i.e., some are more worth protecting than others. If the "system" is at fault, then we introduce the notion of a "usable fiction" into bioethics. The "clinic," the "hospital," or the "system" in short, becomes a fictitious person, as in law, the corporation becomes a legal person. That would be a troubling introduction indeed. It invites "I was only following orders" to become a legitimate bioethical defense.

When a "system" is at fault, moral agency, losing its personal meaning, transfers to decision-makers distant in time and space from the facts on the ground, and, in turn, to the roles they are required to play. Decision-makers too can claim the protection of determinism. To be sure, a system has its own rules, dynamics, and momentum. But, ultimately, it is enacted by persons. If this is denied, ethics is transformed into a problem of design without a designer.

BEYOND GOOD AND EVIL

No matter the dismissal of criminal charges, Dr. Pou and nurses Budo and Landry will have difficulty returning to their careers. Rumor will follow them, eroding reputation and trust. After all, as the common wisdom has it, "Where there's smoke, there's fire." Three years later, the media continue to raise issues posed by the case.

> [If] anyone believed that things have returned to normal for Dr. Anna Pou and her colleagues, CNN and the *Times Picayune* are continuing their pursuit of access to medical records of patients at New Orleans's Memorial Hospital during the harrowing days around Hurricane Katrina. Despite the decision of an Orleans Parish grand jury not to pursue allegations against Dr. Anna Pou and her nurse colleagues in July 2007, both media outlets have continued to assert their right to intrude into patient privacy issues and to foment new controversy where none now exists.[20]

At the same time, friends and colleagues of Dr. Pou established the Dr. Pou Defense Fund. In addition to raising funds to help pay for Dr. Pou's legal costs, it lobbied successfully for legislation designed to protect medical personnel in Louisiana from civil suits and provide a board of professionals to review criminal charges. On June 8, 2008, Governor Bobby Jindal signed the bill, part of a three-piece package, into law.[21]

One of the more obvious consequences of the case of Dr. Pou and nurses Landry and Budo is its likely effect on "first responders." As Dr. Richard Vinroot, who was at the Touro Infirmary during Katrina, remarked, "There are a lot of doctors who have a lot of problems with this [the Pou case]. It's going to have an impact on a lot of people because nobody is going to want to stay for a storm again."[22] Future "good Samaritans" will simply not show up much as physicians in states where there are no "good Samaritan laws" and will tend to avoid getting involved in emergencies for fear of civil suit. When to this is added the risk of criminal prosecution, even good Samaritan laws cannot help. And defending against civil suits and criminal prosecution is always costly no matter innocence or guilt.

Chaos adds another puzzle. Katrina, as we've already noted, was "a disaster waiting to happen." Predictions of a category four or five hurricane were not unknown. Yet, the hospital lacked usable access to a means of evacuation under worst-case conditions, and evidently LifeCare had not sought or found an alternative in the face of those predictions. Preparation of caregivers, and not just at Memorial, for dealing with triage and other likely results of catastrophe was inadequate to the size of the event. Both government and clinic failed to assure basic needs like sufficient emergency power, adequate food, water, medications, and so on. But what chaos also teaches is that preparation is more apt to look backward, to prepare for yesterday's disaster. For example, remembering 9/11, we leave our seaports and subways relatively unprotected while focusing on airport security. The unexpected defeats the standard of care. Aware of this, we may well opt for unconfessed avoidance. Katrina is surely its example. Just about everyone was "playing the odds" that the extreme disaster wouldn't happen on their watch. In defense they might claim that, after all, chaos is the inability to make reliable predictions. In short, can we really know what it means to say, we can prepare for catastrophe?

Finally, there is an almost Kafkaesque quality to Pou's, Budo's, and Landry's experience. They didn't set out to be heroines, but they didn't set out to be villains either. They were just doing what doctors and nurses are supposed to do while many of those around them didn't seem to be doing what doctors and nurses are supposed to do. Suddenly, they are accused of murder and arrested. The affidavit and the warrants, seven months after the event, must have come as a shock even if they knew an investigation was underway.

The Attorney General and the DA apparently do not agree on the law. The experts do not agree on the chemistry; the coroner arrives at a different conclusion. Future good Samaritans will probably abstain. In the public eye, the law seems to punish the heroines. Invert the situation: what if Pou, Budo, and Landry had obeyed the orders to evacuate, leaving the four patients behind? Like others who left when ordered to do so, they would surely have avoided the threat of a criminal trial if not of a guilty conscience.

Among the players, there is near unanimity on the evils of euthanasia. Dr. Pou joins that chorus. As a physician put it,

> While I support passive euthanasia in selected circumstances, I cannot . . . condone active euthanasia. . . . What if I had been in New Orleans and working with critically ill patients? What if my hospital had no electricity? What if we had no means for communicating with the outside world and no expectation of relief? . . . I cannot answer these questions. None of us can truly answer these questions. We do not know what we would do under extreme conditions. If we must make choices, if we must decide who lives and who dies, then how do we do that with compassion and dignity? When we choose who dies (and sometimes we must), how do we minimize the suffering?[23]

Facing catastrophe, we want passionately to return chaos to orderliness. Pou, Budo, and Landry are hostages to that passion. Perhaps Negin, Blanco, and Brown should join them. But orderliness is problematic, which is why I borrow the title of Nietzsche's essay in closing this chapter. We may think to return to a familiar ethical discourse, like the four principles—autonomy, nonmaleficence, beneficence, justice, or the "golden rule"—and thereby to tame catastrophe.

But there is no return. Kenneth Kipnis writes, "In a *medical disaster*, the resources of a health care setting are overwhelmed. Triage helps to solve the problem. In contrast, a *medical catastrophe* occurs when a health care delivery system collapses. The hospital (or any setting where medical care has been provided) has somehow become hazardous to the point where all must relocate to safety."[24] If Dr. Pou's memory is not clouded by what I may call the "fog of catastrophe," then her experience, while extreme, would seem to stir no novel bioethics issues. Palliative care is, after all, a standard treatment. But if she faced a choice between what Kipnis identifies as "forced abandonment" and euthanasia, then our moral common sense offers little guidance. Where there is no third alternative, "Two of the weightiest medical norms are here in collision: the prohibition against abandoning patients and the prohibition against killing them. Where it is impossible to evacuate patients and dangerous and medically futile to remain with them, one of these two norms *must* give way."[25] Both prohibitions remain the norm, but in catastrophe they become inapplicable. Katrina was an omen of the terrorism event and Dr. Pou's experience was emblematic of it. So we are taught the lessons of a moral dilemma that while rare yet increases in likelihood.

With that, we learn that it can happen to us. A colleague whose European experience imports a different consciousness reminds us,

> In one of the Ghettos, the Nazis had there was a "hospital" for children. . . . The physician in charge knew that the Germans were about to evacuate this Ghetto to either Auschwitz or Treblinka. She also knew that they would be sent in cattle cars with no sanitary facilities, barely room enough to stand, no food or water for a few days. After arrival, they were destined to be gassed. She chose to give to each a lethal overdose of, I believe, a barbiturate and then to kill herself. Can anyone condemn this lady or was she indeed doing her best to keep her charges from "harm" and "injustice"? To judge the actions of others is easy when we are in comfort and safety—it is also, in my view, pure hubris. [26]

NOTES

1. Douglas Brinkley, in *The Great Deluge* (Harper Collins, 2006), his comprehensive day-by-day story of Katrina, tells of the many individuals—for example, bus drivers, boat captains, gang leaders, Coast Guard, and Fish and Wildlife personnel. Unlike public and political figures, they will no doubt remain anonymous.

2. "Medical Experts Never Testified in Katrina Hospital Deaths," Drew Griffin and Kathleen Johnston, *CNN*, 8/25/07.

3. "Medical and Ethical Questions Raised on Deaths of Critically Ill Patients," Denise Grady, *NYT*, 7/20/06.

4. "Murder or Mercy? Hurricane Katrina and the Need for Disaster Training," Tyler J. Curiel, *NEJM*, 355, 20, 11/16/06, pp. 2067–69.

5. "But it was on the seventh floor of the hospital where the situation was most dire. Memorial Medical Center leased the floor to LifeCare Hospitals, a separate long-term patient care facility. LifeCare Hospitals is based in Plano, Texas. LifeCare has facilities in nine states and considers itself an acute specialty hospital capable of treating the most complex of cases."

"New Orleans Hospital Staff Discussed Mercy Killings," Carrie Kahn, *National Public Radio* (NPR), 2/17/06.

6. "Dr. Pou further advised T.M. [a LifeCare nurse executive and Director of Education for *LifeCare Hospitals*] that nurses were coming from another part of the hospital to assist Dr. Pou. . . . T.M. was advised that Dr. Pou and these nurses were taking responsibility for the patients and that LifeCare staff should leave." Affidavit, p. 2.

7. NPR, "New Orleans Hospital Staff."

8. Curiel, "Murder or Mercy?".

9. "Good Samaritans or Mercy Killers: And Never the 'Twain Shall Meet," Frank W. Dawkins, November, 2006.

10. Quotes are from "La. Kin Suspicious About Hospital Deaths," *The Associated Press*, 7/20/06.

11. A statement issued by his office (7/19/06) said, "Our Medicaid Fraud Control Unit is mandated by Federal Law, Title 42 CFR, Section 1007, to investigate all allegations of abuse, neglect, or exploitation of the elderly or disabled who receive care from facilities that receive Medicaid funds."

12. "Patient Deaths in New Orleans Brings Arrests," Adam Nossiter and Shaila Dewan, *NYT*, July 19, 2006. There are many types of homicide—for example, justifiable homicide, and negligent homicide. Another option is "manslaughter." The definition that would apply to Foti's comment is "criminal homicide," which is defined as "homicide committed by a person with a criminal state of mind (as intentionally, with premeditation, knowingly, recklessly, or with criminal negligence)." *Find Law*.

13. *Associated Press*, September 21, 2006, citing from an advance release.

14. *LSMS* statement, September 27, 2007, Floyd A. Buras, president.

15. The question before us has to do with whether Dr. Pou foresaw a possible consequence of sedation or intended that consequence to happen. Borrowed from Roman Catholic tradition, modern medical ethics makes use of what is called "double effect." Briefly, it specifies, 1) there is one action with two known effects. 2) One of these effects is good and the other is bad. 3) One foresees both, but intends only the good. 4) The bad is not the cause of the good effect. 5) The good to be achieved outweighs the bad (is undertaken for a proportionate reason).

16. On this point, see the concluding section of chapter 4.

17. Two significant cases on assisted suicide provide important background information on terminal sedation: *Vacco v. Quill* and *Washington v Glucksberg*, decided in June 1997. David Orentlicher commented,

> The pain of most terminally ill patients can be controlled throughout the dying process without heavy sedation or anesthesia. . . . For a very few patients, however, sedation to a sleep-like state may be necessary in the last days or weeks of life to prevent the patient from experiencing severe pain. With this assurance from the medical profession, Justices

> Sandra Day O'Connor, Stephen Breyer, and Ruth Bader Ginsburg wrote in their concurring opinions that the case for a right to assisted suicide had not been made. . . . The alternative of terminal sedation made such a right unnecessary. . . . At first glance, terminal sedation seems consistent with accepted practices. It is appropriate for physicians to treat the pain and other suffering of patients aggressively, even if doing so is likely to hasten death. On closer examination, however, terminal sedation at times is tantamount to euthanasia, or a kind of "slow euthanasia."

"The Supreme Court and Physician-Assisted Suicide—Rejecting Assisted Suicide but Embracing Euthanasia," David Orentlicher, *NEJM*, Vol 337, Number 17, 10/23/97.

18. Affidavit, p. 4.
19. Maurice Bernstein, *MCW listserve*, quoted by permission.
20. Dr. Pou Defense Fund, 10/10/08.
21. Dr. Pou Defense Fund, 7/18/08.
22. "Louisiana Doctor Said to Have Faced Chaos," Christopher Drew and Shaila Dewan, *NYT*, 7/20/06.
23. Robert M. Centor, MD: "Looking for Answers," Roundtable Discussion: "Could Disaster Conditions Ever Justify Euthanasia?" Robert M. Centor, MD; Pennie Marchetti, MD; Roy M. Poses, MD, *Medscape Med Students*, 8(2), 2006. Posted 10/03/2006.
24. "Forced Abandonment and Euthanasia: A Question from Katrina," Kenneth Kipnis, *Social Research* Vol. 74, No 1, Spring 2007, p. 11.
25. "Forced Abandonment," p. 16.
26. Dr. Erich H. Loewy, *MCW listserve*, quoted by permission.

6

SARS

WARNING . . .

> Over the past 15 years, decisions had to be made about how to react to cholera in South America, plague in India, Ebola in Zaire, mad cow disease in Europe, anthrax in the United States, AIDS throughout the world and the annual waves of influenza. In fact, the flu may pose the greatest future risk. There were three influenza pandemics in the Twentieth Century, including the 1918–1919 Spanish Influenza, which killed more than 20 million people, about double the number of people killed during the First World War. A number of experts expect another flu pandemic within a decade.[1]

Terrorism makes for headlines, but nature's terror has no press agents. Epidemic, pandemic, earthquakes, tsunami, hurricane, flood, and famine—the list grows longer. Katrina showed us, once again, how wind and water kill and destroy. We have seen how human beings—willfully or accidentally—can be complicit in nature's destruction. Now we move to another part of the forest, the world of the very small, and how its inhabitants kill, hurt, and terrify us. Nor is human complicity absent. Deliberately or blindly, we are partners of virus and bacteria. Warfare and defense preserve and create deadly members of that world. The things we do or fail to do, the cautions we hear or fail to hear, play their role in accommodating or suppressing the actions of the very small world. Epidemic is invited by contaminated water, open sewage drains, polluted air, crowded slums, failed schools, oppressive poverty, and, not least of all, ignorance and superstition. There is, in short, no excusable determinism embedded in the small world's inevitability.

Choices abound, and where there is choice, there is also responsibility. Bioethics is still on the table.

In this and the next chapter, we will be looking at epidemic and pandemic, at SARS that has already happened and at avian flu that we are warned will happen. Epidemic and pandemic are continuing threats on a planet that teems with life other than our own. Of course, hubris again, we think to eradicate disease and succeed temporarily, at least. Smallpox, polio, and TB come to mind. But soon enough another disease, finding its evolutionary niche, takes their place or a mutation resurrects what we thought we were done with. Efforts to clean house, so to speak, may well make our situation less tenable, less survivable, as with drug-resistant TB. We are indeed part of a "great chain of being," and we scarcely know all the dimensions of our interdependence. There is evolutionary development still to emerge and environmentalism still to be understood that mocks our claims of success and failure.[2]

Notice, by the way, that despite popular anxiety and political "spin," we have not yet reached to bioterrorism in searching out catastrophe. To be sure, the politics and psychology of terrorism drove official priorities and perceptions in Katrina. This made things worse, but in an ancillary manner, so to speak. In the case of epidemic and pandemic, terrorism too is a minority but influential report, but bioterrorism is scarcely present. Of this, more later.

Meanwhile, we need to make sense of infectious disease and its bioethical dimensions. Public health provides geographic distinctions that help us assess the degree of damage and the possibilities of response. Thus, there is outbreak, cluster, epidemic, and pandemic. Below, a rough and ready description:

> Confusion sometimes arises because of overlap between the terms epidemic, outbreak, and cluster. Although they are closely related, epidemic may be used to suggest problems that are geographically widespread, while outbreak and cluster are reserved for problems that involve smaller numbers of people or are more sharply defined in terms of the area of occurrence. For example, an epidemic of influenza could involve an entire state or region, whereas an outbreak of gastroenteritis might be restricted to a nursing home, school, or day-care center. . . . A pandemic is closely related to an epidemic, but it is a problem that has spread over a considerably larger geographic area; influenza pandemics are often global.[3]

With these distinctions in mind, I turn to the SARS epidemic as a model of pandemic.

SARS

SARS (Severe Acute Respiratory Syndrome) is a new infectious disease, a coronavirus-induced pneumonia. While the infection may be present before symptoms appear, sooner or later, its presence is announced by fever, aches and pains, fatigue, headache, shortness of breath, a dry cough. Initially, most of those infected tend to treat it as a common cold. In fact, given the similarity of early symptoms to any number of ordinary illnesses and given a ten-day incubation period, diagnosis is difficult for the clinician as well.[4] By the second week, however, things grow more serious and the symptoms more definitive. Recovery is slow and may take four weeks or more.[5] Like smallpox, SARS is transmitted by face-to-face contact with someone who already has the disease. Personal items like bedding, towels, and dishware that have been used by a SARS patient can also transmit the virus. Antibiotics and antiviral agents are used in treatment. Isolation is necessary for those with the disease and quarantine is necessary for those who have been exposed to the disease, but who may or may not have it. Both isolation and quarantine, however, are difficult to enforce under modern urban conditions.

> In previous centuries, sick and exposed persons were often locked up together in intolerable conditions and received limited medical care. Moreover, quarantine was sometimes applied in an arbitrary and discriminatory fashion, targeting lower socioeconomic classes and racial minorities. The modern concept emphasizes . . . attention to the medical, material, and mental health needs of quarantined persons and protecting fundamental human rights. . . . Quarantine may be applied to individual persons, to small groups, or, in extreme cases, to entire neighborhoods or other geographic districts . . . In the SARS epidemic, persons under quarantine were mostly confined at home and actively monitored for symptoms. In several countries, quarantine was legally mandated and monitored by neighborhood support groups, police and other workers, or video cameras in homes. In other areas, compliance was "requested," but court orders were issued for a small percentage of noncompliant persons.[6]

The first-known case of what was to become the SARS epidemic appeared in Guangdong Province in southern China in November 2002. The patient, a farmer, died. Highly contagious, SARS did not end there. Information about this earliest appearance, however, is sketchy. China did not report the outbreak to the WHO (World Health Organization) until February of 2003. Unwillingness to admit the failures of a troubled health care system evidently caused the delay. A month or so later regular reports to WHO did start to come in after a number of Chinese health care officials and politicians had been fired. Later still, China officially admitted the "cover-up" and apologized for it.

Meanwhile, an American businessman traveling in Southeast Asia on his way to Singapore contracted the disease. Hospitalized in Vietnam, like his farmer predecessor, he too died. Following his death, and an omen of things to come, SARS then appeared particularly among health care workers in the hospital where he had been treated. Ultimately, Vietnam would see sixty-three cases and five deaths. In March, SARS began to show up in Hong Kong (1,755 cases, 299 deaths) and Singapore (238 cases, thirty-three deaths). By the time the epidemic was recognized, it had spread to some twenty-five countries, including major outbreaks in Taiwan (346 cases, thirty-seven deaths) and Canada (438 cases, 375 of them in Toronto, and forty-seven deaths). In the United States, forty-one states and Puerto Rico reported suspected cases of SARS. The total, after analysis, was relatively small: twenty-seven cases and no deaths. Some twenty other nations were affected, although they reported very few cases (in total, eighty-two cases, seven deaths).[7] By and large, Africa, except for South Africa, and Latin America seem to have been spared. For most patients, the disease was serious and debilitating, but they recovered. For some it was deadly. All in all, there were about 8,100 reported cases of SARS and about 10 percent of that global total died.

SARS was all the more threatening because the conditions of modern life made it so. Large mobile populations crowded into urban centers, workplaces, schools, and theaters, or into closed spaces like airplanes, buses, and trains, guaranteed that SARS would spread swiftly. Commercial practices, travel habits, and readily available transportation made SARS an international phenomenon very quickly. Compare, for example, the tempo of the spread of SARS—several months—with that of the 1849 cholera epidemic.

> Cholera, like revolution, had swept through Europe in 1848. Spreading outward from its Ganges homeland, the disease had, in a half-dozen years, visited almost every part of Asia, Europe, and the Middle East. In July 1847, it was in Astrakhan, a year later in Berlin; early in October of 1848 it appeared in London. In the fall of 1848, as in the spring of 1832, cholera poised at the Atlantic. Realistic Americans assumed that this barrier would not long protect the United States. The course of the epidemic was the same as it had been in 1832, except that the Atlantic was now crossed more rapidly, more frequently, and by larger ships.[8]

Apart from its effects on those who got SARS, there was significant "collateral damage," to borrow a phrase from the Vietnam War and made familiar in Iraq II. Not least of all, SARS had disproportionate effects on doctors and nurses. Unlike AIDS that, while a worldwide epidemic, has a slow and deadly pace and a limited mode of transmission, SARS showed us how epidemic and pandemic were likely to appear in today's world. To be sure, the number of cases was small, the death rate low, and the controls effective. At the same time, SARS earned its description, in part at least, as an early warning of what could happen were a more deadly disease or a bioterror attack to occur under modern conditions. The WHO report on "Health Alert Notices to Entering Travelers" is illustrative.

> Combined data from Canada, China (mainland, Hong Kong SAR, and Taiwan), France, Singapore, Switzerland, Thailand, and the United States indicate that approximately 31 million travelers entering these countries received health alert notices. Of these, approximately 1.8 million were reported as arriving from affected areas; this estimate is likely low given the difficulties in tracking travelers and the fact that many airline passengers change planes en route. Inadequate data exist to evaluate the effect of distribution of most of these notices. Mainland China reported distributing 450,000 notices and detecting four SARS cases that may have been linked to the notices (M. Song, China Dept. of Health and Quarantine Supervision and Management, communication to WHO). Thailand reported having printed 1 million notices and detecting 113 cases of illness directly linked to the notices (108 at airports, 1 at a seaport, and 4 at land crossings). Twenty-four cases were suspected of probable SARS: all of which were detected at airports (S. Warintrawat, Ministry of Public Health, Thailand, communication to WHO).[9]

SARS was, in short, a message, but are we ready to hear and respond?

TORONTO

It is not surprising that the largest number of cases was to be found in crowded Asia, often an incubator of infections. About two out of three cases appeared in China alone and one out of five in Hong Kong. The next largest outbreak, however, occurred in Canada, and most of them were to be found in Toronto. With more than two-and-a-half million people, Toronto is one of the largest cities in North America. A center of commerce, it produces about 11 percent of Canada's GDP, topping $127 billion (2005). Extensive reporting on the Toronto SARS experience included postevent bioethical, clinical, and public health assessments, and the results of a three-year study by a special government commission [the "Campbell Report"]. In addition to official reports, a number of research studies investigated how the epidemic was dealt with. Among them were one on preparedness[10] and another on setting hospital priorities.[11] Transparency was a commitment from the outset. Consequently, the Toronto experience is a readily accessible example of the clinical, public health, and bioethical issues that arise in a difficult but manageable epidemic.

Toronto had its first known case of SARS on February 3, 2003. Before it was over four months later, there had been 375 cases and forty-seven deaths. And, before it was over, businesses and schools and places of public assembly like athletic facilities and theaters had closed. The WHO had advised travelers and tourists in particular to avoid the city. Toronto was effectively "shut down." Despite relatively small numbers of infected patients, about 140 per 1 million, SARS was very expensive. With what amounted to a near quarantine of the city itself, opposition from business and political interests to travel alerts and other measures developed particularly since, at one point, the infection rate seemed to be going down. This was a major factor in making what turned out to be a premature and dangerous decision to declare the epidemic over. As was soon demonstrated, Toronto had only seen what came to be called the "first phase."

The first cluster resulted from contact with an infected family member in a Toronto hospital emergency department in February 2003. Three months later, in May, health authorities announced that the outbreak had ended. Public health precautions were relaxed. Very soon thereafter, however, a second and larger outbreak occurred. SARS was back, at first spreading without being detected to patients, staff, visitors, and families at the North York General Hospital. Indeed, hospitals, and not only in Canada, were the source of most SARS infections.

With the second phase, the Ontario health department and the area's hospitals instituted a large-scale program of screening. More than 9,000 people were found to have had contact with actual or potential SARS patients. Others, with symptoms of ordinary colds and other diseases, or no doubt experiencing not unexpected anxiety, turned up to be screened. Of the 9,000, more than 620 were identified as potential cases to be followed and ninety were confirmed. A reporter described his experience of the screening process,

> Today I had a routine visit to a doctor at one of Toronto's largest hospitals. . . . When I got off the bus and went to the small side door that leads to the family practice unit, a sign proclaimed STOP! It redirected me to the main entrance. . . . Ahead of me snaked a long line of people, filling out orange forms. . . . The elevator opens into a parking area, where there's another entrance, another line. At the door, there's a security guard—masked in yellow, no gown—who also squishes some hand-washing liquid from a dispenser and hands me a purple form, asking if I have had fever, cold symptoms, flu-like aches and pains, or if I had visited Southeast Asia in the past 10 days. . . . When I arrive at my doctor's office, my first impression is that it was a leftover police crime scene. Yellow tape is draped over the chairs in the waiting room. A closer look shows that every third chair is clear of the tape. "We have to keep patients more than a metre apart," I am told. . . . "This is probably going to become normal," she told me later as she drew some blood from my arm. . . . At the door where I normally enter the office, the window was covered with a large piece of orange bristol board. The sign read: The Hospital is on Orange Alert.[12]

With a ten-day incubation period and without a reliable diagnostic test, observation and time were the tools for screening, control, and treatment. Home quarantine was the method of choice for those without symptoms; in-hospital isolation for those with the disease. Those who had been quarntined were told to remain at home, have no visitors, wear a mask, wash hands frequently, and sleep in separate rooms. The development of cold-like symptoms and a fever rising above 100.4 degrees Fahrenheit were signs of the disease's likelihood. SARS, like so much else in public health, dealt in probabilities, not certainties.

At North York General Hospital, where "phase two" had been detected, requirements for health care workers were more draconian. Despite the hardship it worked on them, a ten-day work quarantine was imposed on all staff members. When not at the hospital, they were required to stay at home, avoid contact with others in the household, and have no visitors.

North York evacuated its regular patients and stopped admitting new ones. Emergency surgery and ambulatory care were cancelled for seven to ten days after the reappearance of SARS. In about a week, staff members had been trained to deal with the epidemic. Facilities for isolation were set up. Two units able to serve nearly fifty inpatients were converted into SARS wards. The hospital's ICU (intensive care unit) was devoted solely to SARS. Except for hospital staff and recently discharged patients needing follow-up, the emergency department followed a similar policy. A postevent review of the hospital's problems noted,

> Our biggest challenge during the outbreak was insufficient personnel. Most personnel were required at the beginning of each phase and were then needed for approximately 3 1/2 weeks. Although more personnel were recruited, they did not start work for 1 to 2 weeks afteı the initial influx of patients. We required additional nurses, unit managers, infection control personnel, housekeeping staff, ward clerks, and supply stocking and inventory staff. Physicians recruited to manage the outbreak included primary-care doctors, infectious diseases consultants, hospital epidemiologists, public health physicians, emergency department physicians, and radiologists.[13]

"Surge" names the situation when casualties in significantly larger numbers than expected appear suddenly. Of course, emergency departments are prepared to deal with multiple casualty auto accidents, large fires, and localized contagious disease clusters. Given modern specialty and subspecialty, caregivers, for the most part, are not trained for nor do they have experience of epidemic and pandemic. Orders of magnitude change with catastrophes like Katrina or tsunami or with pandemics like the 1918 flu outbreak.[14] Fortunately, SARS was not like these. Yet, its infection rate, the rapidity with which it spread, its potential global reach and its effects on patients, their families, and their communities warranted the international attention it received. Modern medicines, and rapid, widely shared, and relatively adequate information allowed for control. A different disease—Asian flu, as we shall see in the next chapter—or a failure of control would have insured larger and larger numbers of cases and thousands of deaths over a wider and wider territory. SARS, in short, allowed for a manageably scaled process. But it also exposed many of the weaknesses that would also be encountered under catastrophic conditions.

Except for trauma surgeons and emergency department specialists, most physicians and nurses are not trained to deal with mass casualties. Compounding the problem in the United States, emergency departments, trauma centers, and burn units—among the most costly medical facilities—are closing down for lack of adequate funding. Fortunately, Canada's rapid response strategy protected us from the worst effects of the epidemic. Had it not, U.S. casualties would have been far greater and U.S. experience would surely have been far more disastrous.

Toronto was "lucky." SARS's numbers were manageable within the existing hospital system, and the outbreak could be localized using standard public health methods. By contrast, the 1918 flu pandemic was more like Katrina than SARS. Katrina, as we have seen, lost its hospitals, its caregivers, and its police. With an eye to the possibility of more disastrous outbreaks, the 1,200-page Campbell Report, *Spring of Fear*—published January 2007—questioned the adequacy of Ontario's institutional organization.

> The final commission report by Justice Archie Campbell of the Ontario Superior Court . . . said hospitals are dangerous workplaces, like mines and factories, but have inferior workplace safety systems in place. Commission Counsel Doug Hunt told a news conference that hospitals across the province of Ontario were inadequately prepared to control infections and that there was "a systemic, province-wide inadequate acknowledgment of health-care worker safety concerns and preparedness to address them. Justice Campbell found that systemic problems ran through every hospital and every government agency," Hunt said. These included difficulties with internal and external communications and with preparation for an outbreak of a virulent disease.[15]

Interim reports produced by the Commission noted that Ontario did not have adequate provision for communication and planning among the hospitals in the region. For example, "Canada's public health system was hampered by inconsistencies in case definition. . . . The actual definition of a 'case' used by *Health Canada* changed seven times during the SARS outbreak. . . . In particular, these reports (Judge Campbell's two interim reports, 2004, 2005) identified a number of problems . . . including inconsistencies among Canada's provinces, unresolved conflict among [provincial] statutory provisions and general confusion . . . about when and how information may be shared."[16] The import of these comments for the United States, with fifty states and an indefinitely large number of other jurisdictions, each with its own statutory authority, makes the Canadian post mortem frightening indeed.

The final Campbell Report also faulted North York for its inadequate early handling of SARS.

> The outbreak surfaced in February 2003, when a woman from the Toronto area contracted the virus on a trip to Hong Kong and returned home, dying soon after. Her son went to a hospital with an unidentified condition that was later diagnosed as SARS. While waiting for 16 hours in a crowded emergency room, the man transmitted the virus to two other patients, and it continued to spread, the commission's report says.[17]

Even after a patient was free of the disease, clinical problems did not disappear. Events like 9/11, Katrina, and now SARS have a high incidence of PTSD (posttraumatic stress disorder). Its symptoms include flashbacks, nightmares, difficulty concentrating, irritability, etc. Alerted by the research following other disasters, North York established a team to deal with the psychological impact of SARS on both staff and patients.[18] A social worker followed up with discharged patients by telephone. A crisis hot line was available. A psychiatric outpatient system was put in place.

Since SARS was a new infectious disease and so clearly hospital-based, it is not surprising that health care workers were among the largest single group of casualties. More than one hundred suffered the disease, and two nurses and one physician were among the dead.

> Four years after the trauma of the SARS outbreak that claimed 47 lives, Ontario health care workers don't feel a whole lot safer. "On the front lines, there is still not trust in the system. . . . No one will let their guard down," says Ontario Nurses Association President Linda Haslam-Stroud. There is still "a fair bit of concern about the system," adds Ontario Medical Association President Dr. David Bach. But the ONA and OMA, along with others in health care, credit the provincial government with having taken some important steps toward improved safety. . . . The Ministry of Labour has significantly boosted its inspection capability; the independence of the Chief Medical Officer of Health has been increased; money has been allocated for rebuilding public laboratories; and, according to Ontario Health Minister George Smitherman, the province will spend $30 million a year on a new public health agency, which will also include the new laboratory.[19]

DEMOCRATIC SPECULATIONS

For countries like Canada and the United States, conflict often results from the need or claimed need to modify democratic practices in an emergency. Tension, always present, between respect for the dignity of each human being and the need for community safety, if not survival, becomes more complicated and difficult to deal with. Finite resources—time, skill, and wealth—face the problem of best use. In catastrophe, the conflict is intensified. "Best use" acquires a different configuration. Just allocation is guided by principles of disaster triage. A commitment to the autonomy and rights of the individual must make its peace with a utilitarian calculus.

Nondemocratic societies only seem less conflicted. Certainly, they face similar clinical conditions in similar ways. But, they also face their own moral and political problems. Issues of the legitimacy of power and fairness appear in traditional and authoritarian societies, too. The command structure that is needed in the catastrophic event is for them not limited by law or surrendered when the emergency is over. Power and office are permanent possessions of some person or persons, a perquisite or responsibility of birth, status, or position. But this has its price. For example, Ontario authorities needed to issue only twenty-two compulsory quarantine orders. Beijing, on the other hand, had to seal off buildings, use electronic surveillance, and threaten execution in order of deal with SARS.[20] Ultimately, any authority, to be effective, must be and must be seen to be just, or risk subversion and sabotage, as anyone who has lived in a command society can tell you.

Yet, things change. For example, a recent report in the *New England Journal of Medicine* noting the new AIDS treatment program in China reported,

> a striking shift in the government's approach to HIV. . . . Although China's first AIDS cases were discovered in 1989, the government did not publicly acknowledge the existence of a major epidemic until 2001. Two years later, as international attention mounted after the outbreak of severe acute respiratory syndrome (SARS), the government abruptly changed course . . . a national AIDS treatment program was established. The national budget for HIV–AIDS grew from approximately $12.5 million in 2002 to about $100 million in 2005 and about $185 million in 2006. In January 2006, the Chinese Cabinet issued regulations for HIV–AIDS prevention and control, outlining the responsibilities of the central and local governments. . . . The law requires county-level jurisdictions to provide free antiretroviral drugs to poor citizens who need treatment and free consultations and treatment to prevent mother-to-child transmission . . . the statute forbids discrimination . . . in employment, education, marriage, and health care.[21]

Democratic societies are not immune to problems of authority. Decision-making is all too often compromised by influence, wealth, and status. Of course, these are informal and implicit, not official. But, it may be that democracies share more with their authoritarian companions than they may be willing to admit. Indeed, they may experience greater difficulty. Thus, it is one thing to legitimize status and influence by tradition and culture or even by a seizure of power; it is another to allow status and influence to call the tune while denying that they exist. When this is exposed, the democratic problem emerges; authority itself ceases to be believable.

Effective response to catastrophe requires willing participation. Failure to insure public understanding and to provide for fair and objective assessment after the event invites panic. What authoritarian societies attempt to achieve by threat and force, democracies must achieve by trust and its instruments. But, we are forgetful.

> Rare are the calls to prepare the public to respond in their own right. Likely contributing to the neglect of the public's role . . . is the assumption that the general public tends to be irrational, uncoordinated, and uncooperative in emergencies—not to mention prone to panic. . . . As demonstrated by community reactions to the terrorist attacks in New York and Washington, D.C., the power of the public to respond effectively to disasters should not be underestimated. In New York, individual volunteers and organized groups converged on the epicenter of destruction to offer aid and support, despite hazardous conditions and uncertainty about the risks of further attack or structural collapse of the World Trade Center towers. Volunteers responded rapidly and in large numbers to help in search and rescue efforts while professional operations were yet to be put in place.[22]

SARS warns that epidemic does not respect geopolitical or ideological boundaries. Infectious diseases, just like industrialism and market economies, are global phenomena. Consequently, global institutions are necessary to meet global catastrophe. And, in an interdependent world, most catastrophes are or quickly become global. International organizations and international law is monodimensional—that is, a product of the necessary but superficial usage of international bureaucracies. These cannot do the work of bioethics, which must, as it were, sustain moral values while dealing with the realities of culture and tradition. It is no accident, for example, that the Charter of the United Nations had to be complemented a few years later by a Universal Declaration of Human Rights. Nor is it an accident that "nongovernmental organizations" parallel official governments in international affairs.

In a global environment, one size may "fit all" legally, treaties and such, but cannot morally. Social contract societies and secular statute may serve for the West. But for bioethics to deal with epidemic and pandemic, and these are surely global, an anthropological sensibility complements covenant. Culture, custom, and tradition may designate a community's moral agents; for example, "elders" or "shamans" or "clergy." Acceptance of quarantine and isolation may be attached to social roles whose bearers, as it were, "volunteer" the community and its members. Treatment strategies, as we know, vary with religious practices.

Bioethics must also take account of class and caste. Tourism, for example, requires money, time, and interest. Business travel is a function of modern industrial development and a market economy. Both reflect middle-class values and first-world realities. And both contribute to the probability of pandemic. But, a third-world population most often pays the price of pandemic disproportionately. An issue of justice is raised, as neither benefit nor suffering is equitably distributed.

The bioethical agenda keeps growing. Home quarantine and isolation—no visitors including family members, private sleeping quarters—are simply unavailable in most of the world and perhaps even unthinkable in communal societies. Relatively primitive health care in third-world countries and in rural communities cannot cope with new infectious diseases as both AIDS and SARS tell us. A global environment thus forces attention to the ethically appropriate relationship between industrial and developing societies.[23] The connections between doer and done-to, the former privileged, the latter subordinate, evoke a complicated moral situation with, as yet, indeterminate outcomes.[24]

At the same time, the needs of the catastrophic event hint at the globalization of some democratic processes as a precondition of effective response to epidemic and pandemic. Hopeful to that end is the fact that democracy is common political currency if not practice around the world. For example, the vote, for all that it is often corrupted, is symbolic for many peoples of the rightness of social participation. It is not incidental that China, without democratic pretensions but with a growing market economy, acceded to WHO requirements and apologized for "cover-up." Countries ranging across a wide political and social spectrum cooperate with international agencies in reporting cases, broadcasting information, controlling travel, etc. Ironically, disaster thus elevates some democratic values because they are public health necessities. It reminds us too that democracy is a complex idea. No single model exhausts its meaning.

SARS AND THE CANADIAN ENVIRONMENT

As SARS spread to industrialized societies from its Chinese birthplace, it was more likely than not to strike at the middle class and the professional. It is not surprising, and not only because of its origin, that SARS showed up in substantial numbers in highly organized and economically advanced Asian societies like Singapore, Hong Kong, and Taiwan. These communities, however, have moral traditions and legal practices different from those in Western Europe, the United States, and Canada. Autonomy and civil liberties are hardly features of governance in Singapore. Political liberalism is not a major factor in Hong Kong, particularly since it was transferred back to China, nor is it on the agenda in a Taiwan that is still struggling with its identity. Yet, each of these and China too managed well enough to control the epidemic, which suggests that standard public health practices work well in industrialized, market-oriented societies.

Unlike SARS, historic epidemics—for example, cholera, smallpox, plague—more often than not struck the poor in proportionally large numbers of a population. Today, this pattern appears in the AIDS epidemic. In sub-Saharan Africa it decimates whole societies. Among minority populations in the United States, it remains a continuing problem, given the deadly combination of masculine prerogative and religious resistance. As a sexually transmitted disease it also runs afoul of American moralism. These cultural currents are reinforced by minority mistrust of organized medicine as well as the expense of effective treatment. By contrast, SARS was not—or better perhaps, did not become—a mass phenomenon in Asia. In North America, its clinical characteristics together with Canada's egalitarian society and a system of universal health care no doubt contributed to successful control. In short, SARS was different.

With this caution in mind, it is nevertheless instructive to review the issues posed by SARS in Toronto. Fortunately, the University of Toronto's Centre for Bioethics prepared an extensive report on "Ethics and SARS."[25] It identified five paired sets of ethical values: individual liberty and privacy, protection of the public from harm and protection of communities from undue stigmatization, proportionality and duty to provide care, reciprocity and equity, transparency and solidarity. Further, it claimed universal relevance under crisis conditions for these values. Several of these pairs reveal the tension between civil rights and community survival, typical of the distinction between clinical care and public health. Another pair, reciprocity and equity, stressed the community's responsibility to those of whom it expects voluntary compliance with the onerous demands of isolation and quarantine. Proportionality and a "duty to care" called attention to the importance of providing support for those of whom it expects competent professional performance in the face of personal sacrifice and even mortal risk.

Information about the population and geography of an outbreak is needed in order to deal with epidemic. It requires, too, the identification of those who are centers of contagion, beginning with the so-called "index cases." Investigation, in short, is an essential instrument of public health. Privacy and confidentiality become problematic, although this was not a serious problem in Toronto given its tradition of civil liberties. By contrast, in dealing with AIDS in the United States,

> The names of people infected with HIV will be tracked in all 50 states by the end of 2007, marking a victory for federal health officials and a quiet defeat for AIDS advocates who wanted to keep patients' names out of state data bases. . . . The states are bowing to federal pressure so they won't lose money for medications and health services. . . . Some worry that names-based reporting could have the greatest effect on whether minorities and the poor get

> tested and treated because they may be less likely to trust the government to keep their names secret. . . . "After many evaluations of code-based systems, it became clear that those systems do not meet CDC standards for HIV data," said Dr. Timothy Mastro, deputy director of the Division for HIV/AIDS Prevention at the CDC. Diseases such as syphilis, tuberculosis and AIDS already were tracked by patient names, he said, making HIV the exception. . . . "I've not so much changed my opinion as surrendered," said Ron Johnson, deputy executive director of AIDS Action in Washington, D.C.[26]

Race and class bias are not just yesterday's artifacts, as Katrina's Ninth Ward and AIDS demonstrate. Studies of nineteenth-century cholera outbreaks in the United States reveal decided bias toward the poor, the unskilled worker, and the unemployed. In a classic model of blaming the victim, "those people" are accused of inviting disease by their lifestyles and therefore they deserve what happens to them. Still a relevant legal precedent and important as an assertion of federal responsibility, a classic case of prejudice occurred in May of 1900. Nine deaths from bubonic plague were reported in one San Francisco neighborhood. The Board of Supervisors then quarantined the residents. Jew Ho, a grocer, complained, claiming that the quarantine was applied only to Chinese. When local authorities rejected his complaint, he appealed to the federal district court. After review, Justice Morrow wrote,

> this quarantine discriminates against the Chinese population of this city . . . the operation of the quarantine is such as to run along in the rear of certain houses, and that certain houses are excluded, while others are included. . . . The evidence here is clear that this is made to operate against the Chinese population only, and the reason given for it is that the Chinese may communicate the disease from one to the other. That explanation, in the judgment of the court, is not sufficient. It is, in effect . . . discrimination that has been frequently called to the attention of the federal courts where matters of this character have arisen with respect to Chinese. . . . This quarantine . . . is unreasonable, unjust, and oppressive, and therefore contrary to the laws limiting the police powers of the state and municipality in such matters; and, second, that it is discriminating in its character, and is contrary to the provisions of the Fourteenth Amendment of the Constitution of the United States.[27]

Finally, there is the challenge of solidarity, less problematic in Toronto, more so in the United States Isolation and quarantine under modern conditions rely on voluntary compliance. Populations are too large and technology too widely dispersed for a command structure to be effective without the support of the larger community. To some degree at least, triage, isolation, and quarantine rely as much on altruism as on law enforcement; that is, the willingness to accept treatment for some while denying it to others for reasons that defeat personal interest. Solidarity is difficult to achieve in cultures like our own with near absolute commitment to individual choice.

The SARS epidemic was surely a consequence of an interconnected globe. Successful clinical and public health control used traditional public health strategies. These worked because the hospital setting, clinical resources, and means of communication were available. But we have not yet faced pandemic with mass casualties, large numbers of deaths, and fragmented societies under contemporary conditions. So, if it is true that SARS is a warning—the notion with which I began this chapter—then in no small measure it is because it warns us that pandemic is likely and that, lacking an ethics of community, we are not ready to deal with it.

NOTES

1. "Ethics and SARS: Learning Lessons from the Toronto Experience," A report by a working group of The University of Toronto Joint Centre for Bioethics, Toronto, Canada, Revised 13 August 2003.

2. "In this review we consider the new science of Darwinian medicine. While it has often been said that evolutionary theory is the glue that holds the disparate branches of biological inquiry together and gives them direction and purpose, the links to biomedical inquiry have only recently been articulated in a coherent manner. Our aim in this review is to make clear first of all, how evolutionary theory is relevant to medicine; and secondly, how the biomedical sciences have enriched our understanding of evolutionary processes. We will conclude our review with some observations of the philosophical significance of this interplay between evolutionary theory and the biomedical sciences."

"Evolution and Medicine: The Long Reach of 'Dr. Darwin,'" Niall Shanks, Rebecca A. Pyles, *Philosophy, Ethics, and Humanities in Medicine* 2007, Vol. 2:4, 4/3/07.

3. "Epidemic," *Science and Technology Encyclopedia*, McGraw Hill.

4. See "SARS Assessment Clinics Rapid Response to an Infectious Outbreak," Tim Rutledge, et al., *Canadian Journal of Emergency Medicine*, Vol. 7, No. 5/05, pp. 162–67; "Early Diagnosis of SARS: Lessons from the Toronto SARS Outbreak," M. P. Muller, et al, *European Journal of Clinical Microbiology & Infectious Diseases*, Vol. 25, No. 4, April 2006, pp. 230–37.

5. "As in previous reports from other areas, fever was the most frequent initial symptom in our cases. Compared to those previous reports, more patients in our case series initially had diarrhea (31.6 percent vs. 1–19.6 percent). Therefore, according to our observations, diarrhea may be also considered as an early symptom and clue for SARS. In addition, 18 patients had initial symptoms of diarrhea when fever occurred. Gastrointestinal tract should be considered as another important primary infection site of SARS-CoV. A previous study reported the temporal progression of clinical and radiologic findings in SARS patients and indicated that several parameters would become more severe in the second and third week of disease. Our study had similar findings. Although the exacerbation of diarrhea might be due to the use of antimicrobial agents, the diarrhea improved subsequently without their change or discontinuation. Therefore, exacerbation of diarrhea is more likely due to SARS itself. Our study also demonstrates that most patients' abnormal laboratory findings may become more severe in the second week of disease."

"Clinical Manifestations, Laboratory Findings, and Treatment Outcomes of SARS Patients," Jann-Tay Wang; Wang-Huei Sheng; Chi-Tai Fang; Yee-Chun Chen; Jiun-Ling Wang; Chong-Jen Yu; Shan-Chwen Chang; Pan-Chyr Yang [National Taiwan University Hospital, Taipei], *Emerg Infect Dis* 10(5): 818-824, 2004, (CDC), Posted 05/10/2004.

6. "Public Health Interventions and SARS Spread, 2003," David M. Bell; World Health Organization Working Group on Prevention of International and Community Transmission of SARS, *Emerg Infect Dis* 10(11), 2004, (CDC).

7. Data is from the "Epidemic and Pandemic Alert and Response," World Health Organization (WHO), 2003. The numbers are, in all instances, approximate.

8. *The Cholera Years*, Charles E. Rosenberg, University of Chicago Press, 1962, pp. 101–02.

9. "Public Health Interventions and SARS Spread, 2003."

10. "Hospital Preparedness and SARS," Mona R. Loutfy; Tamara Wallington; Tim Rutledge; Barbara Mederski; Keith Rose; Sue Kwolek; Donna McRitchie; Azra Ali; Bryan Wolff; Diane White; Edward Glassman; Marianna Ofner; Don E. Low; Lisa Berger; Allison McGeer; Tom Wong; David Baron; Glenn Berall, *Emerg Infect Dis* 10(5): 771–76, 2004.

11. "SARS and Hospital Priority Setting: A Qualitative Case Study and Evaluation," Jennifer A. H. Bell, Sylvia Hyland, Tania DePellegrin, Ross E. G. Upshur, Mark Bernstein, Douglas K Martin, *BMC Health Services Research*, 4:36, 2004, 12/19/04.

12. In depth: SARS: "The Hospital is on Orange Alert: My visit to the Doctor," Robin Rowland, CBC News Online, May 27, 2003.

13. "Hospital Preparedness and SARS," Mona R. Loutfy et al., *Emerg Infect Dis* 10(5): 771–776, 2004, (CDC).

14. Surge has differentiated functional meanings. Thus,

> Surge capacity: Ability to manage a sudden, unexpected increase in patient volume that would otherwise severely challenge or exceed the current capacity of the health care system;
>
> Surge capability: Ability of the health care system to manage patients who require specialized evaluation or interventions (e.g., contaminated, highly contagious, or burn patients);
>
> Public health surge capacity: Ability of the public health system to increase capacity not only for patient care but also for epidemiologic investigation, risk communication, mass prophylaxis or vaccination, mass fatality management, mental health support, laboratory services, and other activities;
>
> Facility-based surge capacity: Actions taken at the health care facility level that augment services within the response structure of the health care facility; may include responses that are external to the actual structure of the facility but are proximate to it (e.g., medical care provided in tenting on the hospital grounds);
>
> Community-based surge capacity: Actions taken at a community level to supplement health care facility responses. These may provide for triage and initial treatment, nonambulatory care overflow, or isolation (e.g., off-site "hospital" facility).

"Strategies for Patient Care Surge Capacity," Hick et al, *Annals of Emergency Medicine* 44: 3, September 2004, p. 254.

15. "SARS Report Says Ontario Failed Health Workers," Jennifer Kwan, Reuters Health Information, 1/10/07.

16. "Post-SARS: Principles for Design of a Public Health Information System," Elaine Gibson, *Law and Bioethics Report,* Institute for Bioethics, Health Policy, and Law, University of Louisville, Vol. 4, No. 4, Summer 2005, pp. 6–8.

17. "Poor Hospital Practices Blamed for 2003 SARS Epidemic in Toronto." Christopher Mason, *NYT,* 1/10/07.

18. The American Psychological Association ("The Psychological Impact of Terrorism on Vulnerable Populations," *Briefing Sheet,* APA, June 2003) notes,

> Although many in the United States were able to return to a healthy level of functioning following the September 11th terrorist attacks, many Americans continue to experience significant distress. Vulnerable populations, such as women, racial/ethnic groups, and people with prior health and mental health problems, are at increased risk for psychological problems, such as depression, anxiety, and posttraumatic stress disorder (PTSD).

The same description applies to SARS and to other catastrophic events.

19. "Post-SARS: More Protection Needed for Health Care Workers," Ann Silversides, *Canadian Medical Association, Journal,* 176 (4), 02/13/07.

20. Ries, N. M. (2004) *Health Law Rev.* 13, 3–6.

21. "China and HIV—A Window of Opportunity," Bates Gill, PhD, and Susan Okie, MD, *NEJM,* Volume 356, 18, 1801–05, 5/3/07.

22. "Bioterrorism and the People: How to Vaccinate a City against Panic," Thomas A. Glass and Monica Schoch-Spana, *Confronting Biological Weapons,* CID, 34, 1/15/02, pp. 217–23.

23. See, "Meeting the Survival Needs of the World's Least Healthy People (A Proposed Model for Global Health Governance," Lawrence O. Gostin, *JAMA,* Vol 298, No. 2, 07/11/07, pp. 225–28.

24. A dramatic instance is the 1997 debate about the use of placebo-controlled research in third-world countries. The *New York Times* summed it up,

> The experiments . . . involve more than 12,000 pregnant women infected with HIV, the virus that causes AIDS, in Africa, Thailand and the Dominican Republic. The experiments are controversial because only half the women are receiving treatment while the other half are given dummy pills. In the United States, pregnant women who carry HIV receive a course of the drug AZT. . . . But the American regimen is too expensive for third-world nations, and researchers are looking for a less expensive alternative.

("Third-World H.I.V. Experiments Defended," Sheryl Gay Stolberg, *NYT,* 10/2/97).

Marcia Angell, then editor of the *New England Journal of Medicine,* put the issue this way, "Although I believe an argument can be made that a placebo-controlled trial was ethically justifiable because it was still uncertain whether prophylaxis would work, it should not be argued that it was ethical because no prophylaxis is the 'local standard of care' in sub-Saharan Africa. . . . The Declaration of Helsinki requires control groups to receive the 'best' current treatment, not the local one. The shift in wording between 'best' and 'local' may be slight, but the implications are profound. . . . This ethical relativism could result in widespread exploitation of vulnerable Third World populations for research programs that could not be carried out in the sponsoring country. ("The Ethics of Clinical Research in the Third World," *NEJM,* Vol. 337, No. 12, 9/18/97.)

25. "Ethics and SARS: Learning Lessons from the Toronto Experience" (A report by a working group of The University of Toronto Joint Centre for Bioethics), Toronto, Canada, 8/13/03.

26. "HIV Patient Names to be Tracked," *AP*, 4/1/07.

27. *Jew Ho v. Williamson et al*, No. 12940, Circuit Court, N.D., California, 103F.10, June 15, 1900.

7

It Hasn't Happened . . . Yet!

PANDEMIC

Like most middle-class children, I was vaccinated against the usual childhood diseases including, when I was born nearly eighty years ago, smallpox, and then, for the periodic scare about what was called "infantile paralysis" (i.e., polio before Salk and Sabin). I get my seasonal flu shot and read a headline about some new but faraway threat. Later, as a traveler, I had my "shots" for typhoid, hepatitis, tetanus, and whatever else was stirring in the places I was to visit.

In the 1980s, I was introduced to HIV/AIDS and pandemic. A school headmaster at the time, I faced frightened teachers and parents afraid of infection in the classroom. At first, there was AIDS; we thought it was troubling but alien, an affliction of sexual lifestyle or a result of accidental infection. I did my share to fight the initial panic that, around the country, excluded children from classrooms and others from neighborhoods and jobs. I paid attention to what was happening in Africa, Latin America, and the former Soviet Union. As treatments—but not cures—appeared, HIV/AIDS seemed on its way to becoming a chronic disease, at least for people living in wealthy societies and able to afford the tens of thousands of dollars that treatment cost. Although I knew a few young men who had died of AIDS, it was still the "other," as pandemic was the "other." But now, the "other" has grown: some sixty million plus AIDS deaths worldwide and more waiting in the wings. Along the way I learned lessons too about malaria, sleeping sickness, cholera, and TB.

For better or worse, the world of infection has expanded much as our connection to the rest of the world has expanded. SARS and West Nile virus didn't stay over there but came to Europe and North America, too. The media, that not so long ago had reported infectious diseases sporadically and often as a kind of esoterica, began to offer a richer diet of information. We heard of ebola hidden away in sub-Saharan Africa. We were warned—correctly or incorrectly—by Homeland Security that vanquished smallpox might not have been vanquished at all. Addicted to the use and abuse of the latest antibiotics and antivirals, we also heard of new resistant strains of TB. A recent case reads like a modern parable:

> Two hearings last week at the U.S. Congress investigated failures in the case of Andrew Speaker, the 31 year old lawyer from Atlanta who flew to France, Greece, Italy, the Czech Republic, and Canada after being told that he had drug resistant tuberculosis and should not travel on commercial airlines. Health agencies could not prevent him flying, could not locate him on international flights, and were slow to place him on a "no fly" list. The agencies were tardy in notifying the World Health Organization, European countries, and Canada, the hearings found, and a [U.S.] border agent disregarded instructions to stop him. Congressional representatives called Mr. Speaker "a walking biological weapon" and said that if the incident had involved someone with smallpox it could have been disastrous.[1]

In short, the world of public health has really gone public, becoming part of the same world that applauds international trade, the latest technology, and that enjoys a standard of living undreamt of in human history and unreal still for all too many of our fellow human beings.

For many of us, pandemic, a word we had heard but not paid much attention to, entered our vocabularies. To be sure, we knew of epidemic, of contagion, of quarantine, but these were history lessons. I recall, for example, reading Paul DeKruif's *Microbe Hunters* as a teenager—first-rate popular science but unconnected to my world. The list of diseases that we could name and, perhaps, describe, kept on growing. We learned a new connection to other living beings like apes and chickens and cows and pigs and monkeys—only now it was no longer a zoo story but a threat. And, thanks to TV, we became familiar with words like "triage." We began to understand that we truly live in one world and that it has its dark side.

The thought that we westerners too will experience pandemic comes as a surprise. We are used to clean streets, drinkable water, modern sewers, and the like. The dark side even seems an insult to our abilities to command our lives and our environment. Every problem, after all, has a solution. Every disease has its "war" as in a "war on cancer" or "obesity" or what have you. We forget that experience, as John Dewey remarked, is as precarious as it is secure, rich with life's promises and threatened by life's disasters. We forget that famine and flood, earthquake and pestilence have been with us for ages. Thousands of years ago, as Scripture has it, Moses, seeking freedom from Egypt, threatened Pharaoh and his subjects with plague. History tells us that pandemic has decimated armies, whole cities, and even nations, not once, but many times and still does.

Plague betrays its power over our imaginations, becoming a name for all the terrifying things that can happen to us. To be sure, before modern biology and scientific medicine, we might moralize infection, the thought that our evil ways—most often the evil ways of the poor, the criminal, and the "undesirable"—bring with them a deserved punishment. "A pox on you," is after all still a curse. Only in modern times have we moved from theology to causality and from incantation to hygiene. The shift, of course, is not complete. We did not lack for an AIDS theology. We were told that it was God's punishment for the "unnatural" and "ungodly" conduct of homosexuals. More recently, we also heard a flood theology preached to the sinners of the "Big Easy" after Katrina. It, we were told, was punishment for those who rebelled against "God's law." That there was "collateral damage," like dead babies who could neither obey nor disobey God's law, was conveniently ignored.

At the same time, we have become aware of the global dimensions of pandemic. In its fourteenth-century visit, "the Black Death" killed some twenty-five million people, about one-third of Europe's population. Brought from China, still today a reservoir for the disease, it revealed the connection even then, between commerce and infection. Moving through time and space, it searched out its human and its animal victims wherever they might be. As the CDC noted,

> Since China was one of the busiest of the world's trading nations, it was only a matter of time before the outbreak of plague in China spread to western Asia and Europe. In October of 1347, several Italian merchant ships returned from a trip to the Black Sea, one of the key links in trade with China. When the ships docked in Sicily, many of those on board were already dying of plague. Within days the disease spread to the city and the surrounding countryside. An eyewitness tells what happened:
>
> "Realizing what a deadly disaster had come to them, the people quickly drove the Italians from their city. But the disease remained, and soon death was everywhere. Fathers abandoned their sick sons. Lawyers refused to come and make out wills for the dying. Friars and nuns were left to care for the sick, and monasteries and convents were soon deserted, as they were stricken, too. Bodies were left in empty houses, and there was no one to give them a Christian burial."
>
> The disease struck and killed people with terrible speed. The Italian writer Boccaccio said its victims often "ate lunch with their friends and dinner with their ancestors in paradise."[2]

Plague was carried by fleas riding on rats who in turn took it into all the places that rats go. Infected people could easily pass the disease on to others. For some 300 years, plague remained active. While the last major outbreak took place in India and China in 1855, it is still present in parts of East Africa, China, and Southeast Asia. Apparently, however, it has run its course except for small clusters and relatively small numbers; for example, there were about 400 cases in the United States in the last half century and between 3,000 and 4,000 cases annually in Southeast Asia.

Plague had company. Nineteenth-century England and its trading partners around the world saw recurring outbreaks of cholera. The WHO describes it, "Cholera is an acute intestinal infection. . . . It has a short incubation period, from less than one day to five days. . . . [It] causes a copious, painless, watery diarrhea that can quickly lead to severe dehydration and death if treatment is not promptly given." Contaminated water supplies and food and poor or nonexistent treatment of human waste are the primary sources of the bacterium. In his book about John Snow's discovery of how cholera was spread, a classic model of public health journalism, Steven Johnson describes its effects.

> As a matter of practical reality, the threat of sudden devastation—your entire extended family wiped out in a matter of days—was far more immediate than the terror threats of today. At the height of the nineteenth century cholera outbreak, a thousand Londoners would often die of the disease in a matter of weeks. . . . Imagine the terror and panic if a biological attack killed four thousand otherwise healthy New Yorkers over a twenty-day period. Living amid cholera in 1854 was like living in a world where urban tragedies on that scale happened week after week, year after year. A world where it was not at all out of the ordinary for an entire family to die in the space of forty-eight hours, children suffering alone in the arsenic lit dark next to the corpses of their parents.[3]

Cholera appears where water supply is contaminated and sanitation poor. A recent report from Iraq with its damaged infrastructure tells us, "A cholera outbreak in Iraq is spreading, the World Health Organization said Tuesday [9/25/07] with new cases confirmed in Baghdad, Basra and for the first time three northern districts. The number of confirmed cases has now reached 2,116, WHO said. Just a day earlier a WHO official put the number of confirmed cases at 1,652. Eleven people have died of the disease so far."[4]

Despite the effectiveness of public health strategies, epidemic and pandemic continue among us. Some possibilities, like ebola and other animal viruses, are for the moment dependent on animal to human transmission. Appearing in isolated communities, they are thus far expressed in relatively small outbreaks of limited duration. No doubt too, good luck plays a role. But, with AIDS and SARS and, as we shall see, with avian flu, we learn that scientific advances have by no means relegated pandemic to history.

Although the third world and the poor are not immune—when are they ever—SARS told us that advanced industrial societies were certainly vulnerable to pandemic. Unlike AIDS, however, SARS did not offend our Puritan mores. It did not need to wait upon athletes and Hollywood stars to focus attention and billionaires to fund treatment. SARS, thus far, is a disease of the privileged, distributed by market practices in an emerging world economy. In short, we are at risk because of who we have become. "As a number of commentators have noted, SARS exposed the vulnerabilities of our current health care systems and governance structures. . . . Many experts believe that the SARS outbreak was merely a preview of the next flu pandemic that is soon to arrive, possibly from an avian influenza virus."[5]

As the working group of Toronto's Centre for Bioethics warned,

> SARS is a wakeup call about global interdependence, and the increasing risk of the emergence and rapid spread of infectious diseases. There is a need to strengthen the global health system to cope with infectious diseases in the interests of all, including those in the richer and poorer nations. This will require global solidarity and cooperation in the interest of everyone's health.[6]

INDIFFERENCE

If you live in the United States, you're accustomed to annual reminders to "Get your flu shot." If you're over sixty-five years of age, not an infant but under twelve, and don't have an illness that weakens your immune system, you probably did. From time to time, the vaccine will be in short supply and then lines waiting for the injection appear at hospitals, clinics, health departments, physician's offices, pharmacies, and even supermarkets and department stores. It's all very ordinary. The "flu season" usually passes without much remark except for occasional inconvenience.

There have been, of course, exceptions to routine, notably the 1918 pandemic when millions died and the "flu fiasco" of 1976 when millions complained. In the winter of 1976, an army recruit, David Lewis, died of influenza. A few weeks after his death, "swine flu" was named as its cause. Later, studies at Fort Dix would show that some 500 soldiers had been infected, although the cases were mild and recovery easy. Of the nine men who had been tested just after Lewis's death, only four needed to be hospitalized. They too recovered. Except for the soldiers, there were no other reported cases and later on, during South America's winter when flu would be expected, there were no reported cases either. On its face then, things did not seem particularly worrisome.

Nevertheless, there was concern, and it was understandable. Still remembered as the "Great Plague," the 1918 Spanish flu pandemic began among

U.S. troops and spread to Europe when they went overseas. Ultimately, it killed more than 500,000 in the United States and some twenty million or more worldwide; the estimates range from twenty to fifty million. In other words, it killed more people than the "Great War"—World War I—that had just ended. It was thought to have been carried by domestic and wild pigs and was transmitted from person to person. The fact that the 1976 cases affected young, healthy men and bore the name "swine flu" naturally stirred fear of another 1918.

A CDC meeting was called to figure out what needed to be done. As Richard Krause of the National Institutes of Health recalled,

> Sometime in February 1976 a group of . . . influenza experts reached a near consensus that the Fort Dix swine flu was likely to be the source of an imminent pandemic of influenza, perhaps similar to the pandemic of 1918, because Fort Dix virus had the antigenic characteristics of what was thought to be the 1918 virus. . . . Predictably, meetings of the experts were called, and a general sense of alarm prevailed, as well as a sense that something must be done to prevent an epidemic that might be a replay of 1918. All agreed that we needed to enhance national and worldwide surveillance to determine the extent of a possible major outbreak of this virus. . . . [T]he primary question facing us was whether we should quickly prepare a vaccine with the Fort Dix swine flu virus strain and immunize as much of the population as possible.[7]

As it turned out, there were few cases and even fewer deaths. But, what started as a "possibility" became a "probability" for the experts and became a "certainty" for the politicians as the need for decision reached to the upper echelons of government. Finally, in March of 1976, President Ford announced that he would ask the Congress for $135 million in order to "inoculate every man, woman, and child in the United States." The program was begun late the following fall. Very quickly, it appeared that some of those who had been vaccinated developed a side effect, Guillain-Barre syndrome, "a rare, usually reversible but occasionally fatal form of paralysis." About 7 per 1,000, seven times the normal expectation, were affected. By the time the program was stopped in December, some forty-five million people had been vaccinated. The total cost to the government was about $400 million, $90 million of which went to paying damages to those who had developed Guillain-Barre.

FOR THE BIRDS—AVIAN FLU

It's a tricky virus, and we'll never learn all of its tricks. What we do know is that flu virus mutates and adapts quickly, hence the need for ever-new seasonal batches of vaccine. The antibodies that take care of one of its strains are relatively helpless before the mutants that constitute another strain. And on it goes, a fascinating example of viral creativity. Fortunately, most strains for most people cause symptoms reminiscent of a serious cold. While prior vaccinations produce some residual immunity, avian and Spanish flu offer greater resistance to preventive measures.

> Avian influenza virus, strain H5N1, is the latest flu virus with the potential to trigger a pandemic outbreak of flu due to its high lethality in birds and humans. The human population has no known natural immunity to H5N1 because it is genetically distinct from the three flu strains currently circulating in humans (H1N1, H1N2, and H3N2). Bird disease and death from H5N1 have occurred throughout Asia where close interaction between people and poultry has resulted in 114 human cases and 59 deaths from late Dec. 2003 to Sept. 19, 2005 according to WHO. Hundreds of millions of farm birds have been killed throughout Asia in an attempt to control the spread of the virus. New influenza strains like H5N1 arise when two different viruses infect the same animal such as a bird or pig. Since influenza has a segmented RNA genome, individual segments can be exchanged between viruses in a single infected cell creating a new virus. This rare event is called a genetic shift.[8]

But rare events happen! For example, detected in 1997, avian flu appeared in Hong Kong, when several hundred people contracted the disease. But the outbreak was relatively mild. Only eighteen people were hospitalized, and six died. It was transmitted directly from chickens to humans, and young adults had the most severe cases. Above all, it resembled the 1918 pandemic, and so led to the slaughter of some million-and-a-half chickens, after which there were no new human cases.

China and Southeast Asia are most vulnerable to the disease. Chickens and pigs have been a fact of life in the traditional economies of Asian peoples. In rural communities they are found everywhere. A major part of diet and trade, they are in the yard, on the table, and in the local market. To this, we add the appearance of corporate farming now emerging in Asia. For example, following the American pattern, chickens are now "warehoused." Typically, as many as 50,000 birds are raised in a two-story "factory" building. Livestock too are grown in larger and larger numbers and in closer and closer proximity to each other and to human beings. More than 80 percent of the increase in livestock products in Asia in the last decade is accounted for by the industrialization of agriculture. We get some measure of the size of things when we learn that in the first months of 2004, more than 120 million chickens died of flu or of programs to kill infected chickens in order to control the virus.

To date, as far as we know, human-to-human transmission has not taken place. But the virus could mutate—most experts are convinced it will mutate—and, given the numbers and the frequency of contact between livestock, poultry, and humans, the situation is ripe for a species leap. To complicate the matter, the virus also infects ducks and other waterfowl, including migratory birds. So, what happens in China or Thailand or Vietnam does not remain there even if human-to-human contagion does not exist. In short, an avian flu pandemic is likely.

> A pandemic can start when three conditions have been met: a new influenza virus subtype emerges; it infects humans, causing serious illness; and it spreads easily and sustainably among humans. The H5N1 virus amply meets the first two conditions: it is a new virus for humans (H5N1 viruses have never circulated widely among people), and it has infected more than 100 humans, killing over half of them. No one will have immunity should an H5N1-like pandemic virus emerge. All prerequisites for the start of a pandemic have therefore been met save one: the establishment of efficient and sustained human-to-human transmission of the virus. The risk that the H5N1 virus will acquire this ability will persist as long as opportunities for human infections occur. These opportunities, in turn, will persist as long as the virus continues to circulate in birds, and this situation could endure for some years to come.[9]

"[A]though more than 230 million domestic birds have died or been killed, only 251 humans have become ill from H5N1 infection. . . . The current H5N1 virus is apparently not well 'fitted' to replication in humans." However, as the authors of the article conclude, "the virus is always changing and mutations . . . that make it more compatible with human transmission may occur at any time."[10]

POSSIBILITY, PROBABILITY, AND CERTAINTY

Threats are elusive, and media "hype" invites confusion, fear, and ultimately, boredom. I think of my response to warnings about terrorism, of the skepticism and indifference with which announcements by Homeland Security of this or that colored "alert" are greeted. The reasons are not mysterious. We get mixed messages with little assurance of their accuracy or reliability. We learn that according to the "experts," a flu pandemic is a "certainty," and at the same time that it's been around for a decade. We are told that it is a disease of chickens and other birds and only in a minor way a disease of humans, at least thus far. We hear that drug companies are rushing to create a vaccine, that a vaccine is available, that it is or is not very effective, that it will be produced in mass quantities and that it won't be, and that we won't know until the event whether it has helped or not. We get news of the slaughter of chickens by the millions and are then told that wild birds are carriers too and they can't be controlled by slaughter. The threat remains while the event—what kind of event? what kind of threat?—is yet to come. Most of this is truthful to the facts. But delivered in thirty-second bursts of "information," the messages do not give us a coherent picture of what is happening, what is predicted, and what is to be done. We grow used to fearing the "disease" of the week, the latest threat and the latest fad.

Our habit of communicating by "sound bites" is not merely foolish but dangerous. Only when the decision process is transparent can we count on compliance if pandemic demands isolation, quarantine, travel restrictions, and triage. But transparency is not easily achieved. As with the 1976 threat, decision-makers were well intentioned. But their debate went on behind closed doors. We were not informed of their doubts. It could even have been argued that it was better to risk "needless" expense for what turned out to be a nonevent. Instead, the message we heard was certainty. The underlying message was that we couldn't be trusted with the truth.

Preparation for catastrophe is still pretty much restricted to experts and officials.[11] They play the "table-top" games, review the latest research, and generate the policy recommendations. We live with their results. Their assumption is that we need to be fed simple, easily understood bits of information; that is, probabilities become certainties and certainties beget slogans. Consequently, warnings fall on deaf ears. We proceed with our daily routine and strangely, that, it seems, is what we're counseled to do. This advice reinforces a division of labor between those who are the "deciders" and those who are merely their objects. Thus, when advising the public about the "war on terrorism" we are told, "Go about your business." Showing the terrorist that we are not intimidated is the best weapon we have for helping in that "war." Little wonder that skepticism, even cynicism, joins indifference. Health scares like terrorism warnings become only a thing of the moment and are quickly forgotten.

The further consequence is that if and when catastrophe arrives, we will not be ready. In this, SARS seems—but only seems—an exception. It was confined to a limited geographic area and benefited from an intact hospital system. More important, Canada does not have an equivalent to our "inside/outside the beltway" mentality, the alienation of government and citizen. Yet, postevent assessments revealed Canadian weaknesses that, in a less urbane climate and facing a more long-lived event, could have turned a serious outbreak into a catastrophe. As the Pandemic Working Group summed it up,

> One major finding of the JCB [*Joint Center for Bioethics*] research was that people are more likely to accept such decisions [surveillance, isolation, quarantine, triage, etc.] if the decision-making processes are reasonable, open and transparent, inclusive, responsive and accountable, and if reciprocal obligations are respected. Although these principles can sometimes be difficult to implement during a crisis, SARS showed there are costs from not having an agreed-upon ethical framework, including loss of trust, low morale, fear and

> misinformation. SARS taught the world that if ethical frameworks had been more widely used to guide decision-making, this would have increased trust and solidarity within and between health care organizations.[12]

Apart from different magnitudes and sociologies, analysis identifies features of SARS in Canada that do not apply to a catastrophic event in the United States. A brief comparison with Katrina is in point. In the event of an avian flu pandemic, numbers something like those experienced in 1918 could well be involved. A command structure will take over. Communication will probably be reduced to directives. Voluntary compliance—quarantine, isolation, shutdown of public places and businesses, and so on—will no doubt be urged but threat will not be far behind. Denial, resistance, and anxiety are likely outcomes. After pandemic is controlled, undercurrents of resentment will linger along with a good dose of posttraumatic stress disorder. Reconstruction will be slow and sporadic. In short, the SARS lesson is suggestive but limited.

But pandemic hasn't happened yet, just as bioterror hasn't happened yet. And that reinforces our blindness. Of course, authority tries to behave responsibly. Facing public indifference, however, it gets louder, more insistent. Understandable perhaps, this move delivers yet another message, already delivered many times over—people are not competent to deal with catastrophe. Yet, studies of public response to catastrophe—including 9/11 and Katrina—show this to be false to the facts. Nevertheless, the command pattern continues to shape preparation. In short, while the public is expected to trust experts and officials, it is not trusted by them!

In this regard, it is instructive to remind ourselves of some mundane matters. Many of us handle doubt and probability all the time from understanding weather reports to gambling in Las Vegas. The same person who denies his or her mathematical ability calculates prices and, if a sports fan as many Americans are, is quite sophisticated about averages, the odds of winning and losing, the likelihood of finishing with a championship, and the notion that expectations, i.e., probabilities, always include the unexpected. Lately too, TV poker has become a media hit. Latent in all of this is a pedagogical opportunity, but we fail to seize it. Schools and teachers and ordinary citizens are not invited to the "table-top."[13]

Unpleasant and risky events are problematic for all of us, and not just for the "untutored" public. Fear, after all, is a normal and healthy response to danger. But, we tend to exaggerate extraordinary risks and ignore ordinary ones and to exaggerate extraordinary benefits and ignore ordinary ones. In fact, that's what keeps lotteries and medical fads in business. We hear a 10 percent chance of harm differently from a 90 percent chance of benefit, although the arithmetic meaning of these is identical. We worry about the dangers of getting on an airplane more than of getting behind the wheel of a car although we "know" that the plane ride is safer than the car ride. The effort at transparency must account for these psychological features of our response to information, but it seldom does. "Just the facts," which is often the way that transparency is expressed, fails to do the job. We know too that statistical communication is rarely, if ever, neutral. It cannot avoid a point of view. Explicit, hidden, and even nonconscious agendas shape both the content and style of communication. In short, transparency is an achievement and not a formula.

A QUESTION OF JUSTICE

Public health meets pandemic with a menu of familiar strategies: surveillance, mandatory vaccination, evacuation, isolation, quarantine, and triage. These call for radical limitations on personal freedom. In the extreme—say pandemic bird flu, a category 4 or 5 hurricane—we are given two alternatives, obey or suffer. Others, in effect, take control of our lives, briefly if possible, for more extended periods if necessary. Above all, the center of values shifts from autonomy to duty.

In pandemic, as with any catastrophic event, the common good overrides personal preference. Ideally, this loss of freedom can be moralized when, as it were, the common good is internalized, i.e., when, as we say, we "take ownership" of it. The interests of individual and collective are merged. Never entirely realized—the individual and the community are always in tension—many examples exist, e.g., the military unit under battle conditions, the religious order, the athletic "team." We can also find less worthy examples in authoritarian regimes or ideologically rigid associations. Like "individualism," the common good is a two-edged sword. Nevertheless, 9/11, Katrina, and SARS demonstrated our willingness to set personal interest aside for the sake of helping the other. Altruistic French, Germans, and Poles became "rescuers" who, at risk of imprisonment and death, saved Jews from Nazis in occupied Europe. Except under emergency conditions and then only temporarily, we expect, sooner or later, to return to our day-to-day interests and concerns. We are, in other words, the possessors of two distinct moralities. In catastrophe, an "altruistic self" can take over, given the opportunity.

We are not morally ready, except briefly, to treat the community's good as our own and at a cost to our own interests. Our times are against it. Emergency is felt as an intrusion and its moral demands, whatever their merits, are felt as an intrusion, too. In an historic essay, William James struggled with this issue. Ever the philosophic psychologist, he called for a "moral equivalent of war" in recognition—not a little romanticized—of war's appeal to the virtues of patriotism, heroism, and social solidarity. "Martial virtues," he wrote, "must be the enduring cement; intrepidity, contempt of softness, surrender of private interests, obedience to command must still remain the rock upon which states are built."[14] It is not incidental, in this regard, that the U.S. Public Health Service adopts a military pattern of conduct and wears a uniform when mobilizing for catastrophe. Sacrifice joins "enlightened self interest" as a relevant moral category.

To this end, ironically, pandemic may be a moral teacher as hardship is often a moral teacher. However, while social habits may be suspended, they do not vanish. So appeals to the common good arise in a morally ambiguous environment. For example, hierarchies of class and caste continue to shape the content of the common good by specifying who is and who is not included within its moral territory. Less obviously, where social norms like our own allow personal priorities to override social needs, a cloud of distrust attaches to the common good as such. For example, commenting on the case of the noncompliant, TB-infected honeymooner, Wendy Parmet wrote,

> It does seem that [Andrew] Speaker did not react, as we might want him to do. But did he act any differently than many would have under the circumstances? . . . County officials recommended that he not travel to Europe. He ignored that advice. Is that unusual? . . . How many people would follow recommendations to postpone their wedding? Indeed, how many people listen to advice and never go to work or school when they might have the flu? . . . The main problem . . . is not that Speaker's actions are what we would expect of most people. It is that he acted in ways that are perfectly compatible with cultural norms. It is trite but true that in America we admire individual self-sufficiency and rugged individualism. Not only do we admire this "taking care of number 1" attitude, but public health has encouraged it. . . . Even infectious disease policies perpetuate this myth of self-control. We are told to vaccinate our children to protect them. We are told to help ourselves by getting a flu shot. And the federal government provides us with information about how we should prepare to help ourselves and our family in the event of an influenza pandemic.[15]

In other words, we cannot presume that the common good is taken as self-evidently good. Yet, preparation for catastrophe is not so much an intrusion into a way of life but an extension and criticism of it. That is the common message of a time of terrorism and of pandemic. But, our typical preparations for disaster—the periodic gatherings of experts and officials—all too often exhibit the same encapsulization, short-term perspective, and elitism that we find in our efforts at solving other social problems.

Under catastrophic conditions, the common good justifies role-based or functional inequalities. Thus,

> one of the most vexing questions about the just rationing of health care resources is which ethical principle ought to guide decision making—save the most lives (e.g., in fires and floods); save the sickest (e.g., in organ transplant protocols); save the most-likely to recover (e.g., in triage during war); save people who can preserve society (e.g., the Centers for Disease Control (CDC) recommendation during a pandemic). Deciding who can best preserve society means making "social worth" distinctions, which, because they run counter to the instinct for fairness, would ordinarily be considered inappropriate criteria. In the emergency situation of pandemic flu, however, making distinctions on the basis of social worth may be necessary. The hard truth of the matter is that failure to make these sorts of distinctions (giving priority, for example, to doctors, EMS workers, law enforcement personnel, vaccine scientists, firefighters, bus drivers, and sanitation workers) could translate into a high level of injustice accompanied by social chaos, exacerbating an already complicated situation.[16]

But while this view can be defended, it is also vulnerable to the continuing values of the communities in which they are set. Examples of how moralized inequality can mask injustice could be multiplied. The farmer who has seen his flock of chickens and thus his family's economic life destroyed is differently dealt with than the businessman or businesswoman who loses market advantage because of travel restrictions. Little is said about restoring the farmer's capacity for survival. Much is done to help the business get "back on its feet." The first-time homeowner who experiences foreclosure is left to fend for himself or herself. The middle-class family, having a good credit rating, is invited to refinance its home. The poor family, living in crowded quarters, has scant ability to meet the requirements of isolation, just as the lack of transport makes an evacuation order pointless and frightening. The slum dweller without access to clean water and effective sewage hardly benefits from the demands and strategies of the best public health practices. The African American, with a well-tutored skepticism about the intentions of government, transfers his ordinary resistance to the extraordinary condition of disaster. In short, moralized inequalities all too often reflect and perpetuate actual inequalities.

Even within the confines of the event, inequalities can become morally problematic. For example, "first responders" will have access to resources more quickly and more adequately than the general public. And good reasons can be given for this preferential treatment. But, we also identify first responders by status—that is, doctors, nurses, officials, and so on—and thereby provide what may well be an unjustified advantage to a "professional class." Truck drivers—bus drivers in the Katrina situation—and warehouse workers are not ordinarily perceived as "first responders," even when in fact they are or should be.

Scarcity—resources, medicines, food, shelter, transportation—is exacerbated by catastrophe. Access and distribution, a problem of fairness under ordinary conditions, becomes even more problematic when inequalities are moralized by the catastrophic event. Its most dramatic instance is triage. Serving someone with the greatest need is the standard commitment of the helping professions. In the event, this commitment surrenders to a cost and benefit calculation. Need, in other words, transfers from the individual to the collective. Benefit becomes an additive process. Priorities are set by role (e.g., first responders) and utility (i.e., most efficient use of resources). In an interesting reversal of standard moral reasoning that holds that "ought implies can," triage announces, "can implies ought." The moral conflict involved is caught in the following paragraph.

> There are two major options—two moral principles. (a) Those victims for whom we can do the most good could be top priority. That approach rests on the utilitarian principle. (b) Alternatively those with the greatest need could be top priority. That approach is based on the principle of justice. Some with the greatest need are beyond saving. Others with great need can be saved, but doing so will require extraordinary resources. In order to save them, many others with lesser injuries will have to be abandoned. Utilitarians observe that, in some cases, more good can be done in aggregate by targeting those with lesser injuries. Doing the most good for the community of victims would require simply abandoning those who are the worst off. Utilitarians say that that is too bad, but it must be done. Those who would give first priority to the principle of justice reject this option. They would sacrifice the goal of doing as much good as possible. They would let some with minor, but efficiently treatable needs go unattended so that they can do whatever they can for those with the most severe treatable injuries.[17]

Triage is an index of what counts as a moral choice when resource is scarce and survival is at stake. Dealing with it becomes even more difficult when, as is probable in pandemic or catastrophes like the Southeast Asian tsunami or Katrina, hospitals are destroyed, communities are isolated, and supplies are vanishing. Without triage, untreated victims multiply while those with the greatest immediate need benefit. Scarcity increases; fewer resources are available for larger and larger numbers.

When the waters are rising or the number of infected grows, decision is urgent and necessary. At that point, it may almost be said to be thoughtless, automatic, and uncluttered. For this to be morally acceptable, however, the moral legitimacy of the decision process relies on reflection both before and after the event. The moral test of such reflection is its competence—the depoliticization of the expert—and the participation of community voices, i.e., stakeholders. Elected officials partially satisfy the need for representation. But, since they both create and implement policy, they have an "interest" in its success. They also have an interest in making it appear a success even if it is not. The shift from the health of the person to the health of the community—the shift announced by catastrophe—calls for a more inclusive reply at every point to the problem of representation.

Typically, triage, like other emergency practices that are less morally freighted, is treated as if it were morally indifferent, the neutral result of a knowledge-based calculation. Of course, given the either/or of survival, this claim of indifference may well be a necessary fiction. Understood as a technical response to scarcity and need, an objective way of rationing available goods, triage suppresses emotional demands and ignores political and moral context. Or at least that is its claim. But, as with other forms of moralized inequalities, it too can mask interests, institutional prejudices, and justice-distorting cultural norms. For example, as with organ transplant decisions where the probability of "success" is a criterion, social class may be a not-so-hidden feature of decision-making. No doubt, too, retrospective analysis of the catastrophic event will find reasonable grounds for criticism, whatever the choices made. And, no matter how careful and skilled the preparation and the assessment, luck and accident will produce their surprises, too. In one way or another, doing justice in the catastrophic event is going to be problematic.

NOTES

1. "Hearings Highlight Mistakes in Case of Tuberculosis Patient," Janice Hopkins Tanne, *BMJ*, Volume 334, 06/16/07, p. 1242.
2. FAQ, CDC, 2005.
3. *The Ghost Map*, Steven Johnson, Riverhead/Penguin, 2006, p. 85.
4. "WHO: Cholera in Iraq Spreading," Geneva, *The Associated Press*, 9/25/07.
5. "The Plague Fighters: Stopping the Next Pandemic Before It Begins," Evan Ratliff, *Wired Magazine*, 15.05, 04/24/07.
6. "Ethics and SARS: Learning Lessons from the Toronto Experience," A report by a working group of The University of Toronto Joint Centre for Bioethics, Toronto, Canada, Revised 13 August 2003.
7. "The Swine Flu Episode and the Fog of Epidemics," Richard Krause, *Emerging Infectious Diseases*, CDC, Vol 12, No. 1, 1/06. (Reprinted from *Emerging Infections*, Richard M. Krause, Editor, Introduction, pages 1–22.)
8. *Avian Influenza A (H5N1) Fact Sheet*, Federation of American Scientists, Biosecurity and Biodefense, 2005.
9. WHO, 12/05.
10. "H5N1 Influenza—Continuing Evolution and Spread," Robert G. Webster, PhD, and Elena A. Govorkova, MD, PhD, *NEJM*, Vol 355, 21, 2174–2177, 11/23/06.
11. From time to time, efforts are made to improve community participation. Thus, "U.S. officials asked business, health and religious groups on Wednesday to urge Americans to prepare for a possible flu pandemic with steps like storing food and supplies and staying home if ill. Health and Human Services Department

officials met with about 100 representatives of various organizations as part of an effort to convince Americans that the threat from pandemic flu is real and advance preparations can save lives. ["U.S. Government Urges Pandemic Flu Preparations," Will Dunham, *Reuters*, 6/14/07] But, once again, the thinking and planning has been done elsewhere. The community is expected to be relatively passive and uninvolved."

12. *Stand on Guard for Thee, Ethical Considerations in Preparedness Planning for Pandemic Influenza*, November 2005. A report of the University of Toronto Joint Centre for Bioethics, Pandemic Influenza Working Group.

13. It is worth noting that our educational focus is on reading and writing to take "No child left behind" as a message about our priorities. Courses in health and health care are just about nonexistent in our curricula. Science courses—general science and introductory biology, for example—seldom do more than make a nominal reference to how the sciences connect to understanding infectious disease, epidemic, and pandemic.

14. "The Moral Equivalent of War," was published in 1910, Leaflet #27, of the Association for International Conciliation. It was also printed in *McClure's Magazine* [August 1910] and *The Popular Science Monthly* [October 1910]. It was James's effort to find a way to coordinate pacificism and communal spirit.

15. "Quarantine and the Covenant of Trust," Wendy E. Parmet, *Bioethics Forum—The Hastings Center Report*, 6/4/07.

16. "The Coming Pandemic: Ethical Preparedness," Margaret R. McLean, Markula Center, Santa Clara University, 7/07. (From a report prepared for the Santa Clara County Public Health Department on *Ethical Preparedness for Pandemic Influenza*.)

17. "Disaster Preparedness and Triage: Justice and the Common Good," Robert M. Veatch, *The Mount Sinai Journal Of Medicine*, Vol. 72, No. 4, July 2005, pp. 236–41.

8

The Curious Incident of the Dog in the Nighttime

> Colonel Ross still wore an expression which showed the poor opinion which he had formed of my companion's ability, but I saw by the inspector's face that his attention had been keenly aroused.
> "You consider that to be important?" he [Inspector Gregory] asked.
> "Exceedingly so."
> "Is there any point to which you would wish to draw my attention?"
> "To the curious incident of the dog in the night-time."
> "The dog did nothing in the night-time."
> "That was the curious incident," remarked Sherlock Holmes.[1]

Terrorism happens. But save 9/11 and the anthrax event in 2001, there have been no attacks in the United States between then and now, late in 2008.[2] To be sure, there have been threats—most of which turned out to be hoaxes—and arrests of alleged "terrorists" who were said to be plotting attacks but who had yet to mount one. Blocked by a veil of secrecy and thus without reliable information, we are left with doubt and not a little anxiety. But, of course, a terror event is always a possibility!

It's difficult to avoid being skeptical when authorities claim that the absence of attack is in itself evidence of the effectiveness of their efforts. So we are rightly suspicious of reports that seem self-serving. Counterterrorism, after all, is big business. Billions of government dollars are available, reputations are made and broken, and appointed and elective offices are at stake. The temptation to convert threat into fact is very great. The greater temptation, of course, is to believe one's own illusions.

Periodically, we hear from Osama bin Laden or his spokesmen. Their pronouncements seem to reinforce the claims of our government. A cynic might even detect a pattern of mutual support. Terror and counterterror, it would seem, need each other. Without challenging the bona fides of our leaders who may indeed all be "honorable" men and women, we realize that the existence of an "enemy" serves both our needs and theirs.

Fear of terrorist plots was reinforced by Iraq II. Whether mistake or lie, "preemptive war" was justified by the threat of terrorism and the potential possession by terrorists of weapons of mass destruction. In fact, these weapons did not exist, nor, before our invasion, was there a sign of Al Qaeda terrorism in Iraq. But these facts did not dissolve the anxiety that led in the first years after the invasion to public support for the war as an extension of the "war on terrorism." To be sure, there were thousands of casualties, massive destruction, and failing reconstruction. Now, some five years later, attention seems to be shifting to Afghanistan and the Taliban, leaving behind an Iraq, nominally democratic—it has had elections and a parliament—but still struggling with unresolved ethnic divisions and angers. Of course, all of this was and is happening elsewhere and to someone else and not in our backyard. So, except for military men and women and their families, most of us to continue our ordinary lives.

At the same time, bombs in London and Madrid reminded us that terrorism happens and not just in Southeast Asia and the Middle East. As I write (11/27/08) we have news of terrorism in Mumbai. Despite political opportunism in the United States, terror's existence is not in doubt. Uncertainty is our social and political reality. Doubt and fear are inevitable features of living in a time of terrorism. For the terrorist, nearly as much is accomplished by threat and anxiety as by the event itself.

BUT BIOTERROR IS DIFFERENT

Terrorist events live on in our memories. In the mind's eye, we see airplanes striking the Twin Towers, bombs detonating trains and buses, automobiles exploding in the midst of crowds, hostages tortured and beheaded. Given *jihadism*, we see young men and women killing themselves in the act of killing others, and all in the name of the sacred. But the godly legions of radical Islam are not alone. Less vicious and more secular perhaps, "rendition," torture, and "shock and awe" teach us that our claim to virtue is at least questionable.

Terrorism may have strategic credentials—political and religious—but it is inherently nihilistic, as exhibited in its least complicated form in the shootings at Virginia Tech or Columbine. Unconnected to anything other than itself, it is expressive rather than purposive. This reveals terrorism's aesthetic, a genre where the act is an end in itself. The event is theater. The glory of martyrdom plays out on the stage, mingling death's smell with color, and sound.

Even where terrorism pretends to rational ends, it is shaped by the needs of the genre. Whatever its passions or reasons, the event is a message. Bloody and horrifying, terrorism is a way to communicate for those who have little access to power. To be sure, nations including our own are not innocent of terrorism's methods. Hence, "shock and awe" in the opening act of Iraq II. For it to do its job, however, the message needs to be signed much like an artwork is signed. The terrorist may be anonymous, but the event must be authored. Thus, the invention of named groups claiming credit and purpose. Following Aristotle in the *Poetics*, the act must have "a beginning, a middle, and an end." As tragedy, performer and audience experience pity and terror, Aristotle's "catharsis." They are joined in the all-too-human emotions of vulnerability, anger, pain, anxiety, and regret. Unlike the thief and the killer, the terrorist act is deliberately public, even if the terrorist wears a black hood and vanishes into the darkness.

> The apocalyptic imagination has spawned a new kind of violence at the beginning of the twenty-first century. We can, in fact, speak of a worldwide epidemic of violence aimed at massive destruction in the service of various visions of purification and renewal. In particular, we are experiencing what could be called an apocalyptic face-off between Islamist forces, overtly visionary in their willingness to kill and die for their religion, and American forces claiming to be restrained and reasonable but no less visionary in their projection of a cleansing war-making and military power. Both sides are energized by versions of intense idealism; both see themselves as embarked on a mission of combating evil in order to redeem and renew the world; and both are ready to release untold levels of violence to achieve that purpose.[3]

But bioterror *is* different! It is a puzzle for the terrorist art. Lacking theatrical qualities—the sounds and sights of the terrorist act—bioterror fails to satisfy the genre's requirements. Save only nuclear attack, it could be more effective than other methods in its ability to damage and destroy lives and spaces. But, it is subtle, long-lived, and ultimately uncontrollable. A different uncertainty attends it, since we cannot be sure that we face terrorist or nature. And yet, bioterror remains a strategic option. To the aggressor, it offers the power of expanding populationwide destruction, continuing destruction. To the defender, it offers the rewards of preparation without the likelihood of performance, the counterterrorism business again. So bioterrorism can neither be ignored nor expected. It leaves counterterror with the discomforts of uncertainty. It leaves the terrorist with a psychological and tactical dilemma. Little wonder then that bioterrorism is described as "high risk and rare occurrence."

The report on the smallpox vaccination program reminds us,

> Events that involve biologic agents are different from other types of disasters because their emergence is likely to go unnoticed for some time; biologic agents are microscopic and may be more likely to be introduced silently [e.g., through airborne droplets], rather than with explosions, and become evident over time. Also, the fallout from attacks with biologic agents may not remain confined to a specific physical space; in other words, there may not be a "scene" or a "ground zero" and its impact may not be contained but may ripple outward for some time due to contagion.[4]

As the Center for Disease Control [CDC] puts it, "A bioterrorism attack is the deliberate release of viruses, bacteria or other agents used to cause illness or death to people, animals or plants." Spread by air, water, or food, natural and bioterror events are indistinguishable. The casualties exhibit the same symptoms found in epidemic and pandemic. Thus, bioterrorism presents unique investigative puzzles. Public health finds itself with familiar partners like the police and the military doing unfamiliar things. And even where the separation between nature's cause and terrorism's intention is known—as we shall see with the anthrax event—the perpetrator is as likely as not to remain well hidden unless self-confessed, probably unknown and unknowable. Authorship becomes a puzzle.

To this, we may add what is happening in the sciences. Infectious disease can be "weaponized." Using ordinary methods of growing bacteria and viruses, mutated strains can be identified for which existing prevention and cure are ineffective. In nature, flu exhibits this phenomenon; that is, new and often dangerous strains appear regularly without being invited or designed. Given developments in molecular biology, however, the deliberate act becomes more available. It becomes possible to induce and then reproduce preferred mutations or, less elaborately, to rely on their natural occurrence in the rapidly reproducing populations that are characteristic of the small world of bacteria and virus. Exploiting a fecund nature does not require a highly sophisticated biotechnology. Finding or creating it does. Much of this is still a theme for science fiction. That bioterror is not used, however, is more a matter of genre than of capability.

THE DILEMMA OF PREPAREDNESS

Bioterror events are rare, so we have only minor and often failed attempts to look at. Thus, in 1984, the Rajneeshee Indian cult contaminated several salad bars with salmonella. There were 750 cases of poisoning, forty were hospitalized, but there were no deaths. In the 1990s, Japan's Aum Shinrikyo made numerous attempts to spread anthrax, botulism, Q fever, and ebola, but failed. And, as we shall see, the 2001 anthrax event in the United States, while finally identifying an alleged perpetrator in 2008, remains something of a mystery. With bioterror, unlike guns and bombs, preparation and defense become puzzles of scientific and technical capability. Of course, we try to prepare. But we will not know how effective our preparations will be until they are tested in the event and probably well after the event is identified for what it is.

Our most ambitious attempt to be prepared has been the Department of Homeland Security. Gathering together intelligence, military, law enforcement, and emergency response agencies, it reflects the apparently sensible idea of integrating the instruments of protection that will be needed in the event of catastrophe. But, as Katrina showed, putting agencies together does not assure effective performance. Institutional competition does not disappear. As was evident in SARS, conflicting priorities, work habits, and vocabularies serve to delay rather than facilitate response. A tragic and relatively simple example emerging from 9/11 mirrors part of the problem. Police and fire departments tried to coordinate their efforts, but they were defeated by difficulties of communication and command. Differences of mission and style handicapped performance despite the heroism of individual police and firefighters. Airport security, after more than seven years of trying, is still vulnerable. Efforts to inform the public about "threat level" are met with indifference and even gallows humor.

Another instance of the problems of preparation is "BioShield," a multibillion-dollar program to stock America's emergency "medical cabinet" with the drugs and vaccines needed to respond to a bioterror event. The project was announced by the president with the usual fanfare, "We will rally the great promise of American science and innovation to confront the greatest danger of our time." The reality turned out differently. As the *New York Times* reported,

> So far, only a small fraction of the anticipated remedies are available. Drug companies have waited months, if not years, for government agencies to decide which treatments they want and in what quantities. Unable to attract large pharmaceutical corporations to join the endeavor, the government is instead relying on small start-up companies that often have no proven track record. . . . "The inept implementation of the program has led the best brains and the best scientists to give up, to look elsewhere or devote their resources to medical initiatives that are not focused on biodefense," said Michael Greenberger, director of the Center for Health and Homeland Security at the University of Maryland.[5]

"Table-top" exercises are another way to prepare. Borrowing from the military, these exercises bring together federal, state, and local government officials and technical experts. Scenarios are described, roles are assigned, and possible responses to the problems they pose are played out. One of the first of these exercises was "Dark Winter" in June of 2001. A mock National Security Council is charged with dealing with a suspected Iraqi bioterror attack on the United States. Thousands of cases of smallpox are reported across the country. Vaccines run short; the health care system is overwhelmed; and government loses credibility. Three hundred thousand casualties are predicted, and it is estimated that one-third of them will die. Cases are also diagnosed in Canada, Mexico, and England. Inevitably there are food and medical shortages.

The comments of several senior participants are revealing,

> "We are used to thinking about health problems as naturally occurring problems outside the framework of a malicious actor. . . . If you're going against someone who is using . . . disease . . . quite rationally and craftily, but using it toward an entirely unreasonable and god awful end—we are in a world we haven't ever really been in before."
>
> "This was very revealing to me—that there is something out there that can cause havoc in my state that I know nothing about, and for that matter, the federal family doesn't know a whole lot about either."
>
> "This was unique . . . [you know] that you're in for a long term problem, and it's going to get worse and worse and worse and worse and worse."[6]

The exercise—before 9/11, Katrina, and Iraq II—exhibited our technical and logistic unreadiness. At the same time, an existential gap also appeared—"we are in a world we haven't ever really been in before"—a gap that improved technical and quantitative responses could not close. Moral and political values need as much attention as hardware. Failure to account for these predicts the failure of preparation for the event. Yet, they seem a luxury when buildings are falling, people are dying, and the wounded are bleeding. Preparation, therefore, tends to focus on "realistic" problems. So it is likely that moral values will be ignored or dismissed. At the same time, effective decision-making relies on trust, honesty, and respect, i.e., on moral values.

Another illustration of the problems of preparedness was the smallpox vaccination program announced by the president in December 2002. Well before that date, there had been continuing review by CDC and state health officials of the likelihood of a smallpox or anthrax event. Responding to 9/11 and the anthrax attacks, the decision was made to vaccinate both military personnel and civilians. The Department of Defense [DoD] succeeded in vaccinating more than 600,000 by the end of 2004. The civilian program told another story.

Conceived as a three-phase program, the initial goal was to vaccinate 500,000 health-care and public-health-response teams in a thirty-day period. Following that, other "first responders"—up to ten million—were to be vaccinated. By 2004, a "new vaccine," if ready, would be offered to the general public. The program was nominally supported by health care agencies around the country. But as the word spread, there were doubts about the safety of the vaccine, about the accuracy of the data, and about the costs to already limited budgets. Individual hospitals, caregivers, and local government officials were interviewed in January and February 2003 and

> people involved in the program reflected a wide array of commitments and feelings. They included commitment to doing what was needed to protect the public's health, confusion and suspicion about the rationale for the program, confidence in the usefulness of vaccination, concern about the vaccine's safety and about the potential loss of wages because of non-life-threatening but important post-vaccination symptoms, and criticism of or worry about the reluctance of many public health and health care workers to be vaccinated. The net results of individual and institutional concerns were hesitation and low participation among public health and health care workers and great variability in hospital participation.[7]

There were just too many unknowns. The vaccination program as such was a puzzle to those asked to participate, neither a typical public health program nor a research study. The unfamiliar territory of biodefense contributed added uncertainty. Of course, the program appealed to our patriotism. At the same time, the program increased our anxiety. The "top-down" design of the project from policy to planning to implementation stirred the resistance of caregivers and institutions that are typically jealous of their independence and that ordinarily make their own decisions. In any event, as of 2004, less than 50,000 caregivers had been vaccinated, about 10 percent of the original goal. Little has changed since then.

Bioterror threatens the basics of survival: food, water, and air. Each of these also has symbolic meaning; for example, the communal meal, baptism, and so on. Bioterror threatens death and, as worrisome, incapacity, lingering debility, and a continuum of risk and doubt. In short, it is the stuff that makes for nightmares. Bioterror preparedness is thus marked by hesitation and ambiguity. Nor are we confident in the abilities of those entrusted with the responsibility. Certainly, periodic shortages of flu vaccine and the failures of Katrina signal a lack of competence. Doubt can only increase when natural events are added to the complexities of hostility and defense. But, even if major bioterror events have not happened—one puzzling incident, anthrax, in nearly a decade—we cannot be confident that they will not happen. Thus, the dilemma of bioterrorism: it rarely happens, so why an investment of scarce resources; it can happen, so do we dare not to make that investment. Caught in a utilitarian dead end, we turn to smallpox, the bioterror event that has not happened and anthrax, the bioterror event that has happened. But I do not know if looking at them helps or hinders us in dissolving the dilemma.

A SCRATCH OF PREVENTION

In 1967, the World Health Organization (WHO) led a global campaign to eradicate smallpox. In 1980, declaring that the disease had been eradicated, it recommended stopping all vaccination in all countries. Two "reference laboratories" were established, one in the United States, the other in the Soviet Union (now Russia). Early on, there were allegations that the latter was continuing its biological warfare program. In 1980, a Russian biologist, Ken Alibek, who had worked in its Offensive Biological Weapons Program, claimed that the USSR had begun production of the smallpox virus. But, as with so much about bioterrorism, the evidence was circumstantial and inconclusive.

Since the dissolution of the Soviet Union, there have been rumors that its troubled military establishment might sell its bioterror weapons or its technical knowledge to so-called "rogue states" and to bioterrorists. But, rumor is not fact and allegation is not evidence. As Jeffrey Drazen wrote, "At the present time, there is no way to know. If smallpox virus is in the hands of bioterrorists, then it could be a threat. If all the infective virus is securely held by responsible authorities, then it is not a threat. Since virus stocks cannot be tracked with accuracy, it is impossible to know the answer to this important question."[8] We do know that the United States is building a stock of vaccines and trying to develop more effective ones. But the control and security of smallpox agents remains problematic. Thus,

> The World Health Organization (WHO) . . . delayed for at least four years any decision on when to destroy the world's last known stockpiles of smallpox. . . . [It] reaffirmed a previous commitment to getting rid of the remaining stockpiles but agreed to postpone any decision on when this should happen until its 2011 meeting. . . . A previous 2002 deadline for destroying smallpox had been waived . . . until new vaccines or treatments for smallpox were found, after the United States said it would keep stocks on hand to combat any re-emergence of the disease.[9]

The optimism of the 1980 announcement has vanished. The CDC described the situation, "In the aftermath of the events of September and October, 2001, the U.S. government is taking precautions to be ready to deal with a bioterrorist attack using smallpox as a weapon."[10] And the AMA noted, "We are not expecting a smallpox attack, but the recent events that include the use of biological agents as weapons [i.e., the anthrax event] have heightened our awareness of the possibility of such an attack. . . . At this time we have no information that suggests an imminent smallpox threat."[11]

Smallpox is highly contagious. It is spread by contact from person to person, by bodily fluids, or by contaminated bedding or clothing. Consequently, cremation is advised and potentially contaminated objects should be burned.

Smallpox has a long, terrifying, and destructive history. For centuries, until the discovery of a vaccination by Edward Jenner at the end of the eighteenth century, smallpox, along with cholera, and plague, afflicted nations across Europe and Asia. It was brought to the New World by European explorers. Reportedly, the British tried to use the disease as a weapon in the French and Indian Wars, allegedly giving smallpox-contaminated blankets and goods to Native Americans. Whatever the cause—explorers' contagion or military tactics or both—smallpox decimated the native population.

Today, bioterror security focuses on possibility rather than likelihood. As an article in the *Journal of Homeland Security* put it, "The probability of a smallpox bioterrorist event remains unknown, but the level of vulnerability of the United States population makes the threat too great to ignore. The U.S. smallpox vaccination program ended in 1972, leaving 119 million Americans fully susceptible to the disease in 2003. The 157 million U.S. citizens vaccinated before that time likely have little or no protection left."[12]

As recently as the first half of the twentieth century, major outbreaks of smallpox occurred: New York City in 1901 had 1,960 cases and 400 deaths; Denver in 1921, more than 900 cases and nearly forty deaths; Kansas City, also in 1921, about 950 cases and 160 deaths; and Detroit in 1924, 1,500 cases and sixteen deaths. Responding to a threatened epidemic, in a remarkable demonstration of public health's increasing sophistication, and with communitywide participation, six million out of New York's seven million people were vaccinated in 1947.

> Local public health officials got everyone involved in the process, including federal and state governments, aid organizations such as the Red Cross, drug companies and community organizations. They also used education and volunteerism rather than coercion. . . . "The health department really respected the public's need to know," said Dr. [Judith] Leavitt. "They weren't putting a spin on it. And the public health infrastructure was in extremely good shape and gained support by reaching deep into community networks." Physicians working at the time credit the success of the effort to something much simpler: fear. Smallpox hadn't been seen in New York City in decades, but it was still a very real threat and endemic in much of the world. "People were terrified," said James Dick, MD, who was a resident at the Postgraduate Medical School and Hospital in New York.[13]

While outbreaks have long since ceased, individual cases still appear. For example, two deaths from smallpox were reported in Birmingham, England, as a result of laboratory accidents. Recently, "A two-year-old boy spent seven weeks in the hospital and nearly died from a viral infection he got from the smallpox vaccination his father received before shipping out to

Iraq, according to a government report and the doctors who treated him."[14] Given the rarity of its occurrence, doctors and nurses lack familiarity with the disease. And given its contagion and our vulnerability, in-hospital contacts are a likely source of such cases. But prevention, too, has its price. For example, recent research reported that, depending on the particular vaccine strain that is used and the health of the population involved, estimates of deaths from a mass inoculation program range from as few as ten to as many as 1,000 per million.[15]

DETECTIVE STORY—THE ANTHRAX ATTACK

On September 18, 2001, just seven days after the Twin Towers fell, an assistant to Tom Brokaw, a well-known commentator at NBC, opened a letter that contained a white powder. A week later, she noticed lesions on her chest. These spread over much of her body, and in the next weeks she also developed headaches and experienced general malaise. Fortunately, after treatment with antibiotics, she recovered. But that was just the beginning.

Over the next five weeks, similar letters were received by an ABC producer. Her seven-month-old son, while visiting his mother at work, developed the disease. After treatment, he too recovered. Cases of cutaneous anthrax also appeared at CBS, the *NY Times*, and the *NY Post*. Two workers at American Media Incorporated were diagnosed with inhalational anthrax although both were initially misdiagnosed—one as suffering from meningitis, the other from pneumonia. Of the two, Robert Stevens, a sixty-year-old, died, the "first bioterrorist casualty of this millennium" as Paul Rega in *The Bioterrorism Response Manual* puts it.

After the attack on the media, the scene shifted to government. In mid-October, a letter was sent to Tom Daschle, then the Senate Majority Leader. While the Senator did not see it, a number of staff members had handled the letter in transit. Twenty-eight of them tested positive for exposure to anthrax. Workers in the D.C. post office were infected, and two of them died of the disease. Federal office buildings were closed for inspection and decontamination, among them the regional postal center, the Senate Office Building, the Supreme Court, and the CIA. Since the letters came from the New York City area, albeit with false return addresses, the Postal Service tested some 200 facilities along the East Coast for anthrax contamination. Before the attack ended some 10,000 people had been placed on antibiotics as a precaution. Ultimately, there were twenty-one anthrax cases and three deaths; a small number to be sure, but a costly and frightening massive event.

Anthrax is caused by a spore-forming bacterium, *Bacillus anthracis*. People can get it from contact with infected animals, wool, meat, or hides. There are three types: skin (*cutaneous*), lung (*inhalation*), and digestive (*gastrointestinal*). In its most common form, anthrax causes skin ulcers, fever, and fatigue. Up to 20 percent of those infected will die if untreated.[16] Anthrax can be "weaponized."

> It is possible to . . . manipulate the anthrax spores to increase the likelihood that contact with them will result in infection. For example, spores can be "milled" into a size (one to three microns) that would make them optimal for inhalation deep into the lungs. . . . Spores can also be coated with an electrostatic powder so that they do not clump easily and fall to the ground quickly; these spores would then be more easily aerosolized (dispersed into the air). It is also possible to genetically engineer the anthrax bacteria before they turn into spores to make them more resistant to antibiotics. . . . One of the major problems with anthrax spores is the potentially long incubation period. . . . Exposure to an aerosol of anthrax spores could cause symptoms as soon as two days after exposure. However, illness could also develop as late as six weeks after exposure. . . . Typically, symptoms appear at about seven to ten days after exposure. . . . In the current situation . . . there will be opportunity for anthrax spores to come into direct contact with the body of the person and thus, cutaneous anthrax will likely occur . . . Spores contained in the envelope can also become aerosolized should the envelope be jarred or opened or mechanically manipulated. Individuals in close proximity who then inhale these spores could then develop inhalational anthrax.[17]

Efforts began immediately to determine if the anthrax used was in fact weaponized and to learn the identity and motivation of the terrorist[s]. The FBI, Homeland Security, and the U.S. Postal Service as well as local law enforcement joined the investigation. The message accompanying the white powder was printed in uppercase letters. The first note, dated with obvious purpose, September 11, was typical,

> YOU CAN NOT STOP US. WE HAVE THIS ANTHRAX. TAKE PENACILIN [SIC] NOW. DEATH TO AMERICA, DEATH TO ISRAEL, ALLAH IS GREAT.

An FBI profile was developed. A special task force, Amerithrax, was established and was still at work in 2008. Some commentators claimed that the anthrax used had been weaponized and that therefore its production required a high degree of technical skill and sophisticated laboratory resources. Others said it was a standard infectious agent and easily accessible. Still others suspected cover-up. The FBI concluded that the spores "bore no special coatings to increase its deadliness and no hallmarks of a military weapon."[18] An Iraqi connection was officially denied. Inevitably, Al Qaeda was invoked, but this too was denied. The perpetrator, it was believed, worked alone and was "homegrown."

Steven Hatfill, an Army biodefense researcher, after months of investigation, was neither charged nor cleared, but he was identified as a "person of interest"—a relatively new and troubling violation of due process. As a result, he lost his job and no doubt his career. In a suit he filed against the FBI and the Justice Department he maintained that the leaks had "destroyed his reputation." Nearly seven years after the attack, after thousands of interviews and more than 5,000 subpoenas, the perpetrator remained unknown. Then, in June 2008, "The Justice Department announced . . . that it would pay $4.6 million to settle a lawsuit filed by Steven J. Hatfill. . . . The settlement, consisting of $2.825 million in cash and an annuity paying Dr. Hatfill $150,000 a year for twenty years, brings to an end a five-year legal battle."[19] In August 2008, the FBI announced that it had identified the perpetrator, Bruce Ivins. In November, the FBI documents were released,

> A federal court on Tuesday unsealed documents that shed new light on why F.B.I. anthrax investigators spent years pursuing the wrong man. . . . Search warrant affidavits said that Dr. Hatfill filled prescriptions for the antibiotic Cipro, the preferred drug for treatment of anthrax, two days before each of the mailings of anthrax-laced letters in September and October 2001. . . . The documents report that Dr. Hatfill spoke of serving in a Rhodesian military unit accused of starting an anthrax epidemic in 1979, told an acquaintance that it would take a "Pearl Harbor-type attack" to awaken the United States to the bioterrorist threat and kept an anthrax simulant in his apartment. In August [2008], after the suicide of another researcher who worked at the same Army laboratory, Dr. Bruce E. Ivins, the F.B.I. said it had concluded that Dr. Ivins alone had carried out the anthrax attacks. . . . The Justice Department then made public search warrant affidavits laying out circumstantial evidence against Dr. Ivins, including symptoms of mental illness, late hours in the laboratory before the mailings and genetic evidence linking the mailed anthrax to a supply in his laboratory. But no definitive evidence has tied Dr. Ivins directly to the letters or to the site of the mailings in Princeton, N.J., and many of his colleagues and friends have said they do not believe he committed the crime.[20]

We know the cause and its outcome. We know its casualties—ultimately seventeen people got sick and five died. We know the millions of dollars spent and still being spent on the investigation. We know it has not been repeated. Finally, we know that,

> the anthrax letters were an entirely new phenomenon. Despite hundreds of anthrax hoaxes prior to 2001, this was the first time that actual anthrax spores had been used in the United States. These anthrax incidents were small-scale, and apparently intended to frighten rather than kill large numbers of people. Since 2001, there have been many hoaxes, where the senders claim to be sending anthrax, but actually enclose a harmless white powder. In many cases, hazardous material teams respond to the hoaxes at great cost to the public and disruption to businesses. The U.S. government has allocated billions of dollars to detecting and combating anthrax and other biological weapons. The U.S.

> Postal Service has installed machines across the country that monitor the mail for anthrax or other biological agents. Some experts argue that the huge U.S. spending on bioterrorism is out of proportion to the threat.[21]

Finally, we know that bioterror is still rare, still costly, still frightening. And since Dr. Ivins committed suicide, much about the anthrax attack remains a mystery.

A QUESTION OF RESPECT

Skill and technique are not enough. Catastrophes, natural or intentional, have a moral dimension. Participation, competence, and fairness are prerequisites for effectiveness. Without them, trust vanishes. And with that,

> the trust of the general public in government and government's ability to protect the public's health is a critical requirement for responding to bioterrorism (or any other public health threats) . . . people's trust in government must be handled with great care, but it is an essential requirement for effective communication; people are less likely to panic and more likely to participate constructively during an emergency if they believe they can trust government agencies to provide accurate and timely information.[22]

In turn, participation, competence, and fairness rely on respect for persons. Instrumental to and symbolic of respect is truthful communication. Where security does not permit, brief and honest explanations during the event and full disclosure after it preserve the moral standing of democratic authority. "Need to know" may be an appropriate category in an emergency. Indefinitely extended emergencies, however—like a "war on terror"—cannot help but stir suspicion. When communication becomes propaganda, usually with a nod to democratic piety, a type of deafness develops. No message, true or false, gets through. Anger and resentment are typical when we find out we've been lied to, fooled, or manipulated. And we do find out. We become "noncompliant" as the clinician has it. Resistance and covert sabotage follow.

Moral values, already challenged in the harsh climate of natural catastrophe, become even more problematic when terrorism, real or threatened, enters the scene. As in the case of Dr. Pou, but on a larger scale, moral values become ambiguous. Public health, clinical medicine, law enforcement, and the military seem to speak a common moral language. In fact, they do not. Moral dissonance increases. For example,

> An attack with biological agents would put into motion two major and divergent systems (in addition to many others): public health, which attempts to deal with consequences and spread of infectious disease, and law enforcement,

> which targets the commission of a crime implicit in a deliberate introduction of a biologic agent. In the anthrax attacks of 2001, differences between public health and law enforcement became apparent. These included different investigative approaches (inductive versus deductive respectively), evidentiary standards (scientific versus legal), and communication objectives. Public health tried to share complete and accurate information with the public in a timely manner, while law enforcement sought to disclose little or nothing pertaining to an investigation in order to maintain the integrity of a potential legal case.[23]

To the different traditions and missions of clinical medicine, public health, law enforcement, and the military are added problems of institutional organization and practice. To be sure, in the midst of catastrophe, civil authority and public health adopt a command structure too—witness the provisions of the Emergency Powers Act. But, this move is understood as conditional and temporary. The courts adapt to the exigencies of the situation, that is, the temporary waiver of due process as in quarantine and statutory specifications for delaying appeals, as in the seizure of property. Authority, however, is still exercised by democratically designated offices and officers. Law—constitutional and statutory—establishes a continuum of legitimacy.

Police, military, and caregiver do share national loyalties and patriotic values, although with different emphasis and passion. Like the general public, they can be targets of limited and distorted information. On the ground, however, they are less likely to be fooled by claims that are demonstrably untrustworthy. Caregivers, for example, know the inadequacy of supply, the effectiveness of medication, the level of preparedness, and the like. A disconnect between truth and promise becomes visible. The consequence is likely to be alienation from each other and from authority as such. Deteriorating morale is one index of the situation. Anomie and amorality are another.

Duties are compromised or ignored. The military's experience in Vietnam provides the moral lesson. Illustrative is the debate about the role of caregivers and soldiers in situations of "rendition" and "interrogation."

> The role of military medicine in these abuses merits special attention because of the moral obligations of medical professionals with regard to torture and because of horror at health professionals who are silently or actively complicit with torture. Active medical complicity with torture has occurred throughout the world. Physicians collaborated with torture during Saddam Hussein's regime. . . . Physicians in Chile, Egypt, Turkey and other nations have taken great personal risks to expose state-sponsored torture. Military personnel treating prisoners of war face a "dual loyalty conflict." The Geneva Convention addresses this ethical dilemma squarely: "Although [medical personnel] shall be subject to the internal discipline of the camp . . . such personnel may not be compelled to carry out any work other than that concerned with their medical

> . . . duties." By this standard, the moral advocacy of military medicine for the detainees of the war on terror broke down.[24]

In a time of terrorism, public health, the police, the military, and clinical medicine acquire new missions. Police powers that historically supported efforts to control disease become dominant. Forensic needs—what counts as evidence and how it is used—compete with public health investigation. For the military, the priority is identifying and defeating an enemy. Healing, culpability, and victory are three guiding ends-in-view. They can and do conflict. The need for security competes with transparency. Law enforcement requires confidential investigation, health care requires respect for autonomy and informed consent, and military strategy requires sacrifice, disinformation, and secrecy. Not least of all, each institution has its own history, tradition, practice, and language. So, while the common good is surely at play in all four, style, procedure, mean, and proximate ends are radically different. In a time of terrorism, they intersect. Respect for persons under the conditions we have described is fragile indeed. Making moral sense is inevitably problematic.

NOTES

1. *The Memoirs of Sherlock Holmes* (1893), "Inspector Gregory and Sherlock Holmes in 'Silver Blaze,' New York, Doubleday, pp. 346–47.

2. In a computer search for "bioterrorism, anthrax, and smallpox," the typical reply was: "No incidents met the search criteria." 1/1/2004–12/31/2006, Worldwide Incident Search, National Counterterrorism Center. The Center was established by Presidential Order in 2004. Its most recent report (*Report on Terrorism*, April 2008) noted,

> Approximately 14,000 terrorist attacks occurred in various countries during 2007, resulting in over 22,000 deaths. Compared to 2006, attacks remained approximately the same in 2007 while deaths rose by 1,800, a 9 percent increase from last year's number. As was the case in the previous two years, the largest number of reported attacks and deaths occurred in Near East and South Asia. These two regions accounted for about 87 percent of the 355 casualty attacks that killed 10 or more people—only 45 casualty attacks occurred in Africa, East Asia & Pacific, Europe & Eurasia, and Western Hemisphere. . . . As was the case in 2006, most 2007 attacks were perpetrated by terrorists applying conventional fighting methods such as bombs and weapons including small arms. However, technology continues to empower terrorists and effective methods of attack are offsetting countermeasures against terrorism. Terrorists continued their practice of coordinated attacks including secondary attacks on first responders at attack sites with uniquely configured weapons and other materials to create improvised explosive devices (IED), including the introduction of chemical IEDs in 2007. (pp. 9–10)

3. "American Apocalypse," Robert Jay Lifton, *The Nation*, 12/8 and 12/22/03.

4. *The Smallpox Vaccination Program*, Institute of Medicine, National Academies Press, 2005, p. 290.

5. "Bid to Stockpile Bioterror Drugs Stymied by Setbacks," Eric Lipton, *NYT*, 9/18/06.

6. On June 22–23, 2001, The Johns Hopkins Center for Civilian Biodefense Studies, in conjunction with The Center for Strategic and International Studies, The ANSER Institute for Homeland Security, and The Oklahoma National Memorial Institute for the Prevention of Terrorism, held an exercise at Andrews Air Force Base in Washington, D.C. entitled "Dark Winter." The first such exercise of its kind, "Dark Winter" was constructed as a series of mock National Security Council (NSC) meetings in reaction to a fictional, covert smallpox attack in the United States. "Lessons of Dark Winter," Tara O'Toole, MD, MPH, Thomas Inglesby, MD, Johns Hopkins Center for Civilian Biodefense Studies.

7. *The Smallpox Vaccination Program*, Institute of Medicine, National Academies Press, 2005, p. 44.

8. "Smallpox and Bioterrorism," Jeffrey M. Drazen, *NEJM*, Vol. 346, No. 17, 4/25/02, pp. 1262–63.

9. "UN Again Delays Destruction of Smallpox Virus," Reuters, 5/18/07.

10. *CDC Fact Sheet*, 2006.

11. *AMA FAQ*, 2005.

12. "The Threat of Smallpox: Eradicated but Not Erased: A Review of the Fiscal, Logistical, and Legal Obstacles Impacting the Phase I Vaccination Program," Holly Myers, Elin Gursky, Georges Benjamin, Christopher Gozdor, and Michael Greenberger, *Journal of Homeland Security*, February 2004.

13. "Smallpox 1947: 'People were terrified,'" Victoria Stagg Elliott, *American Medical News*, 6/23/03.

14. "Soldier's Smallpox Inoculation Sickens Son," John Schwartz, *NYT*, 5/18/07.

15. "Frequency of Adverse Events after Vaccination with Different Vaccinia Strains," Mirjam Kretzschmar, Jacco Wallinga, Peter Teunis, Shuqin Xing, Rafael Mikolajczyk, *PLoS Medicine*, Volume 3, Issue 8, e272, August 2006, pp. 1341–51.

16. *DHHS*, 2003.

17. "Anthrax, Frequently Asked Questions," *AMA*, 2005.

18. "Anthrax Not Weapons Grade, Official Says," William J. Broad, *NYT*, 9/26/06.

19. "Scientist Is Paid Millions by U.S. in Anthrax Suit," Scott Shane and Eric Lichtblau, *NYT*, 6/28/08.

20. "New Details on F.B.I.'s False Start in Anthrax Case," Scott Shane and Eric Lichtblau, *NYT*, 11/26/08.

21. "Anthrax Attacks and Bioterrorism, WMD 411," *Monterey Institute's Center for Nonproliferation Studies*, updated November 2006.

22. *The Smallpox Vaccination Program*, Institute of Medicine, The National Academic Press, Washington D.C., 2005, p. 101.

23. *The Smallpox Vaccination Program*, p. 296.

24. Review and Opinion, "Health and Human Rights, Abu Ghraib: Its Legacy for Military Medicine," Steven H. Miles, *Lancet*, Volume 364, Number 9435, 8/21/04.

9

Sword of Damocles?

THE PANDORA PROBLEM

"It's a puzzlement," as the king says to Anna in *Anna and the King of Siam*. And so it is. Bioterrorism is a sometime thing. Yet the literature of bioterror is plentiful and the budget, growing. Nearly all of what we hear is phrased in the rhetoric of inevitability. No doubt, opportunism, cupidity, and self-delusion are at work. Terrorism is, after all, useful to political animals like presidents and presidential candidates. Bioterrorism is particularly useful because it is invisible, elusive, and mysterious. But genuine public health concerns and good science are also at work. Thus, the theme of this penultimate chapter—an attempt to figure out what's going on behind the disconnect between what has happened and what, it is said, will have to happen.

Threats deal in futures; in this instance, ominous futures. With these, like Pandora, we have loosed the dilemmas of prediction. We "know" that whatever materializes will not be good for us. Even the shadows, especially the shadows, are an affliction.

Event or not, bioterrorism is a political, psychological, and economic reality. Like nuclear bombs, it is a "weapon of mass destruction." Yet, the bioterror events we know about have been small in scale and few in number. Standing against this history is conviction: "Not if but when," is the message we hear. So, we prepare, lest needless death and destruction follow! But, in the absence of the event, what does preparation mean?

Given the thinness of the bioterror record, we turn to natural events like plague and pox. They tell us that the cost of being unprepared is measured in thousands of needless deaths and even larger numbers of serious but nonfatal casualties. Preparation, however, has its casualties too, and we are already on that road. 9/11 and Iraq II are, as we say, incidents in a "war on terrorism." Reacting, we have already reshaped our laws and practices, and ourselves as well, in order to prepare for a next strike. Moreover, in trying to undo what has been done in the name of counterterrorism, we meet yet other unknowns, some of which might also be deadly. The prospect—indifference, defense, or reconstruction—is dizzying, and the risks of preparing or of failing to prepare are unavoidable. The Pandora's box is open, and the evils released.

A METAPHYSICAL PLOY

Anxiety may be defined in a rough and ready way as fear without an object, like the ghosts that haunt us when passing a graveyard in the night. As the National Institute of Mental Health describes it,

> People with generalized anxiety disorder go through the day filled with exaggerated worry and tension, even though there is little or nothing to provoke it. They anticipate disaster and are overly concerned about health issues, money, family problems, or difficulties at work. Sometimes just the thought of getting through the day produces anxiety.
>
> Unlike clinical anxiety, bioterror feeds on existential anxiety, as it were, "normal" anxiety.
>
> I grasp myself as threatened or as vulnerable; but unlike fear, anxiety has no direct object, there is nothing in the world that is threatening. This is because anxiety pulls me altogether out of the circuit of those projects thanks to which things are there for me in meaningful ways; I can no longer "gear into" the world. And with this collapse of my practical immersion in roles and projects, I also lose the basic sense of who I am that is provided by these roles. In thus robbing me of the possibility of practical self-identification, anxiety teaches me that I do not coincide with anything that I factically am.[1]

With terrorism, vulnerability becomes a standard condition. Pandora's ills do not vanish with the dawn. Terrorism is thus a psychosocial fact, a state of being. Even falsehood—the existence of weapons of mass destruction in Iraq for example—remains a "truth." The terror event, echoing in our consciousness, our feelings, and our behavior, is quickly recalled by a photograph, a sound, a word. There is neither victory nor defeat, only the rhythmic flow of highs and lows. Will the next shopping bag hold a bomb, the next stranger be a holy suicide? And there *will* be another shopping bag, another stranger! "Ordinary" acts of terrorism, dramatic, sudden, and tangible, dissolve anxiety into fear and anger, allowing for analysis and defense. When the event ends, however, anxiety returns. Suspicion lingers, doubt lingers, worry lingers.

Unlike bombs and guns, bioterrorism is born in doubt itself, builds on doubt itself. The threat is a weapon as deadly in its way as infection in its way. Will the next letter contain anthrax; the next breath, pox? Is the white powder nature's pandemic, terrorism's weapon, or only talcum? Biology takes time, and only time will allow answers if answers there be. Little wonder, then, that while fear accompanies terrorism, existential anxiety is a particular asset of bioterrorism.

As early as 1999, The Commission on National Security warned, "Taken together, the evidence suggests that threats to American security will be more diffuse, harder to anticipate, and more difficult to neutralize than ever before. . . . There will be a blurring of boundaries: between homeland defense and foreign policy; between sovereign states and a plethora of protectorates and autonomous zones."[2] In short, we will live with radical uncertainty for the foreseeable future. One way to manage it, as chess and bridge players know, is to consult the probabilities and then adopt a determinist strategy. We plan for a future as if it will happen in a certain way; we opt for inevitability of one kind or another. Philosophy provides an example too in Vaihinger's "philosophy of as if."[3] Inevitability is a relief. Unfocused fear, now focused, becomes a problem of reason. But the risk of this either/or strategy is win or lose. Fortunately, there's always another chess game, another deal. Terror's choice, however, is life or death. Its world, now reduced to certainty, is no longer a strategic hypothetical. We learn to believe in its reality. Ironically, we then call it realism.

With inevitability, the rituals of an obsessive patient become available. A patient is relieved by the diagnosis; an anxious student, by the grade. Insisting on closure no matter the situation is a way to control events. Even where closure is a pipe dream, it is preferable to uncertainty. So too, with the citizen, the politician, and the expert. With inevitability—bioterror will happen—relief becomes a collective and not just a personal phenomenon. Counterterrorism finds its footing, able to read backward from a *certain* future to present tactic. Table-top exercises like "Dark Winter" or "Blue-Advance-02" mirror this "reality." In the process, what started as an "as if," a surrogate for the actual, becomes the actual. Real-time policies and programs follow.[4] We have made the metaphysical move, and now we know what to do. We adopt an information policy that feeds on secrecy and deny the applicability of international law. We distort the truth for the sake of a greater truth, and we agree to command authority, a fit companion to determinism. We choose different budget priorities.

Nor is this only a philosopher's speculation. John Mueller reminds us,

> For the past five years, Americans have been regularly regaled with dire predictions of another major al Qaeda attack in the United States. In 2003, a group of 200 senior government officials and business executives, many of them specialists in security and terrorism, pronounced it likely that a terror-

> ist strike more devastating than 9/11—possibly involving weapons of mass destruction—would occur before the end of 2004. In May 2004, Attorney General John Ashcroft warned that al Qaeda could "hit hard" in the next few months and said that 90 percent of the arrangements for an attack on U.S. soil were complete. That fall, *Newsweek* reported that it was "practically an article of faith among counterterrorism officials" that al Qaeda would strike in the run-up to the November 2004 election. When that "October surprise" failed to materialize, the focus shifted: [to] a taped encyclical from Osama bin Laden, [who,] it was said, demonstrated that he was too weak to attack before the election but was marshalling his resources to do so months after it.[5]

Mueller concludes, "The massive and expensive homeland security apparatus erected since 9/11 may be persecuting some, spying on many, inconveniencing most, and taxing all to defend the United States against an enemy that scarcely exists."[6] And yet, reading these sentences, something in us says, it hasn't happened yet!

To the anthrax attack and the minor bioterror events we have already noted, we can add a few historic instances of agroterror, another type of bioterror.[7] In the Civil War, Union troops attempted to infest Confederate food supplies with harlequin bugs. In World War I, German agents attempted to infect livestock being shipped from the United States to Europe with anthrax. Thousands of horses were killed, although the effort had little strategic effect. Mau Mau in Kenya and Tamil Tigers in East Asia attempted agroterror, too. Chemical attack is not unknown. Mustard, phosgene, and chlorine gas were used in trench warfare. In World War II, the Japanese tested anthrax, cholera, plague, and typhoid on Chinese prisoners. Thousands died. But the bacteria could not be weaponized and so could not be used effectively on the battlefield. Both the United States and the Soviet Union, beginning in the 1940s, developed elaborate bioweapons research programs, although they were not used in World War II, Korea, or Vietnam.

Taken all together, the record is one of sporadic attempts and minimal results. Nevertheless, bioterror enjoys elevated status in today's terrorism talk, not least of all because of the use of chemical attack by Saddam Hussein against the Kurds after Iraq I and the alleged threat of weapons of mass destruction in the run-up to Iraq II.

THE PRECAUTIONARY PRINCIPLE

Past performance, as my stockbroker reminds me, does not guarantee future results. Tomorrow, in other words, bioterror may no longer be a minor report in the terrorism story. The risk of deliberate pandemic grows. As SARS demonstrated, world travel, large concentrated populations, and technical skill make us more and more vulnerable to infectious disease. As it were, we need to think about building bioterror's levees against the possibility of bioterror's "100 year storms." Unfortunately, biodefenses are disease-specific, so we cannot know what kind of levees to build.

We may not know right away if pandemic flu or "mad cow disease" or what have you is a terrorist attack or a natural event. Indeed, we may never know. So, even if the metaphysical ploy were to satisfy our "quest for certainty," we would still experience methodological messiness.

How then, might we proceed? Facing the likelihood of environmental disasters, a 1998 conference developed the Precautionary Principle. While not intended for the purpose, it suggests a helpful way of looking at counterterrorism and at bioterror in particular. Summing it up,

> An international group of scientists, government officials, lawyers, and labor and grass-roots environmental activists met January 23–25 at Wingspread in Racine, Wisconsin to define and discuss the Precautionary Principle. . . . "The process of applying the Precautionary Principle must be open, informed and democratic and must include potentially affected parties. It must also involve an examination of the full range of alternatives, including no action." Thus, as formulated here, the principle of precautionary action has 4 parts:
>
> 1. People have a duty to take anticipatory action to prevent harm.
> 2. The burden of proof of harmlessness of a new technology, process, activity, or chemical lies with the proponents, not with the general public.
> 3. Before using a new technology, process, or chemical, or starting a new activity, people have an obligation to examine "a full range of alternatives" including the alternative of doing nothing.
> 4. Decisions applying the Precautionary Principle must be "open, informed, and democratic" and "must include affected parties."[8]

The Precautionary Principle is, if you will, a *cautionary* principle and particularly valuable in warning of the risks of counterterrorism. Its core values—participation, information, and transparency—set democracy's limits. Secrecy, command authority, and surrender to technical expertise have been our methods of choice. Given the psychology and politics of a "war on terrorism," the Principle's openness, to "examine a full range of alternatives," is too easily dismissed.

Under attack—real or imagined—the public mood shifts from anxiety to fear and anger. Finding the villain becomes an emotional priority. So resistance to the Principle's guidelines is understandable. Understandable too is our reliance on building a culturally isolated counterterror structure. Religious, educational, economic, and voluntary institutions play little role in counterterror policy-making.[9] For example, death and dying need a religious perception as much as a clinical one. Typically counterterror coopts them, as with "embedding" reporters in military units during Iraq II.

Tactical security becomes an excuse for propaganda and censorship. Community organizations like schools and churches can play many roles—communication, morale, emergency services—but are reduced to serving as agents of a command structure. In short, in our thinking and planning for the reconstruction of community in the face of a terror event, we yield to a counterterrorism strategy narrowly conceived: defense against and victory over a terrorist enemy. Even where consulted, the community is seduced, adopting the same counterterror narrowness of perception that is our counterterror style. Thus,

> Despite the rarity of bioterrorist incidents, multi-billion dollar programs have been underway over the past three years in the U.S.—well before the anthrax cases appeared in 2001—for "preparedness" against bioterrorism. Many public health organizations—including the Centers for Disease Control and Prevention (CDC), other units of the U.S. Public Health Service, and numerous county and state departments of public health—are engaged in these programs. Institutes to study bioterrorism have been established and schools of public health are being encouraged to set up core curricula on the topic. . . . A huge, coordinated program involving law enforcement and national security agencies has been undertaken, with enormous implications for public health and medical care services.[10]

The Precautionary Principle expects us to consider taking no action at all. This provides benchmarks, telling us where and how far any given option might take us and where and how far a "war on terror" has already taken us. The null hypothesis alerts us to the fact that inquiry cannot be confined to technical rearrangements and readjustments, i.e., to tactics and strategy. Counterterror's ends-in-view and the values that shape them need their criticism as well.

Finally, the Principle urges the use of our imaginations—thinking "out of the box" as we say. But sadly, even this imperative becomes standardized, formulaic. All too often solutions to the problems of identifying and choosing among alternatives are dictated by an illusion of self-evidence. As often, experts tend to think within the limits of their professional reality, to turn determinism into technological determinism. Surgeons see surgical solutions, psychiatrists see psychiatric ones, and soldiers see military ones. Institutions, in other words, generate their own realities and with them the perceptions of their members.

Ideas, options, and solutions emerge from the reality we perceive. So, enriched perception and democratic decision-making require an inclusive array of choices; as it were, a community of choices. Effective inquiry is dialogic. It requires diverse voices. Even in crisis, perhaps particularly in crisis, no institution, class, or competence can claim a monopoly of wisdom. By way of extending this thought, a brief look at criminal justice, homeland security, and the "law of nations."

Criminal Justice

Terrorism appears in a multinational environment. It is a strategy of what are called "nonstate actors" and "rogue states." That latter is a dubious label since membership in that category depends on who is making the designation. The United States will have one list, Iran another, China yet another, etc. Responsibility for counterterror may be assigned to any of several institutions—criminal justice, the military, international organization, or to some newly invented structure. Each choice reflects a society's moral and political values and, not least of all, its public mood.

On its face, terrorism looks very much like a crime. Thus,

> A biocrime is similar to an assault crime, except, instead of a gun or knife, the weapon is a pathogen or a toxin. In the U.S., acts of bioterrorism are federal crimes. . . . The numerous hoaxes that are biocrimes include white powders found in letters that proclaim the presence of anthrax, and threatening notes claiming ricin contamination of baby food. . . . Nonetheless, a hoax is also a crime, and the physician should not discard any evidence simply because material appears innocuous.[11]

Canada, Australia, and most European countries turn to the police—often using special police intelligence units—and the courts to deal with terrorism. Terrorism, so perceived, is dealt with according to democratic norms and protected by democratic controls—due process, reliance on evidence, public trials, etc. Of course, it would not do to romanticize criminal justice. The police have been known to violate civil liberties, exhibit bias toward ethnic minorities, and take legal, and moral, shortcuts. Courts are not immune to the prejudices of judges and prosecutors. Both can be driven by political pressure and, not least of all, by public opinion.

Nevertheless, by choosing criminal justice, counterterrorism aligns itself with a society's cultural practices. This move minimizes the temptation to treat terrorism as mysterious and alien. To that extent, it reduces the force of existential anxiety that, as we have seen, reacts to the unknowable threat. Citizen participation, as in jury trials and the ballot box, reduces the chance of panic and encourages voluntary compliance with a catastrophe's needs.[12] Thus, reports after the London bombings (July 2005) marveled at the calm of the wounded caught deep underground in darkened subway trains waiting for rescue. No doubt, memories of the Blitz allowed a certain cultural stoicism.[13] With the second, but failed, attempt a few weeks later and with the failed effort in London and Glasgow more recently (July 2007), the Brits, like the Israelis, "normalized" terrorism, as it were. As much a matter of policy as of sociology, Britain's new prime minister made the turn to criminal justice explicit,

> When terrorists tried to blow up civilians in London and Glasgow, Gordon Brown, the new British prime minister, responded in his own distinctive way. What had just been narrowly averted, he said, was not a new jihadist act of war but instead a criminal act. As if to underscore the point, Brown instructed his ministers that the phrase "war on terror" was no longer to be used. . . . Brown, it seems, has concluded that the war rhetoric employed by Blair was divisive, threatening social peace between communities in Britain, and counterproductive. . . . In other words, the Brown approach would be the approach of serious crime fighters around the world these days—community policing in which mutual trust is the cornerstone of crime prevention.[14]

In short, counterterror was not an encapsulated phenomenon. Not even the outbreak of "mad cow" disease in Great Britain stirred the angst of bioterrorism.[15]

To be sure, all is not smooth and easy. Criminal justice, public health, and clinical medicine have different purposes. Often complementary, these can result in conflict (i.e., between care and detection, between cure and punishment). But these three are civic institutions with relationships that have historic precedent. In a time of terrorism, however, their tasks expand. "Police power," ordinarily an instrument of public health, moves toward the investigative and punitive functions of criminal justice. Public health and clinical medicine acquire a new partner with an old name. At the same time, all three continue to live in the same neighborhood. In principle and law, albeit at times in uncomfortable practice, they share democratic values. Terrorism forces change, of course, the development of uneasy but functional relationships that yet draw on a common history and tradition.[16] The alienation invited by terrorism, however, is by and large avoided.

Homeland Security

No other Western democracy has adopted America's institutional dualism. With the PATRIOT Acts (2001, 2006), the United States deliberately isolated its citizens from a counterterrorist program that lives in its own fenced-off territory. A mélange of police, military, health care, and political agencies, Homeland Security emerged after 9/11 as its own cultural and social reality. Public information was reduced to signals like this or that colored alert or to generalized warnings that lacked meaningful content. Not least of all, this dualism invited the reaction, "it's not my business." Signals without consequent events invited skepticism. In short, the "war on terrorism" and its counterterror agency is peculiar to the United States.[17] It legitimizes security practices that are constitutionally dubious and political gamesmanship that often functions as a scare tactic. At the same time, it subverts traditional democratic institutions.

The British, while they have their own problems with civil liberty, are not loath to challenge the strategies of the United States. For example,

> Two prominent British counterterrorism figures have criticized the United States for what they described as its overly militaristic approach to fighting terrorism. . . . One of the experts, Stella Rimington, a former director general of Britain's domestic intelligence agency, said in an interview published over the weekend that she hoped the next American president "would stop using the phrase 'war on terror.'" The British have been critical of Guantánamo Bay, secret detentions and the denial of habeas corpus to terrorism suspects in the United States, but the intrusion on individual privacy here is greater than in America. Surveillance cameras are ubiquitous—in subway stations, in residential neighborhoods, on highways. . . . The surveillance has probably made the British citizenry the most watched in the world, outside of Singapore. . . . Britain has approached terrorism more as a criminal matter than as a military one. In contrast to the United States. . . . Britain has prosecuted suspects in all the major terrorist attacks in the country since 2005. And it has achieved a 90 percent conviction rate, Mr. Macdonald, head of the Crown Prosecution Service, said in a speech on Monday. "The trials," he said, have been "absolutely grounded in due process and pursued with full respect for our historical norms and our liberal Constitution."[18]

The rhetoric of American counterterrorism is revealing. For example, the National Strategy for Combating Terrorism announced by the White House in September 2006 read,

> Our strategy also recognizes that the War on Terror is a different kind of war. From the beginning, it has been both a battle of arms and a battle of ideas. Not only do we fight our terrorist enemies on the battlefield, we promote freedom and human dignity as alternatives to the terrorists' perverse vision of oppression and totalitarian rule. The paradigm for combating terrorism now involves the application of all elements of our national power and influence. Not only do we employ military power, we use diplomatic, financial, intelligence, and law enforcement activities to protect the Homeland and extend our defenses, disrupt terrorist operations, and deprive our enemies of what they need to operate and survive. We have broken old orthodoxies that once confined our counterterrorism efforts primarily to the criminal justice domain.[19]

A "war on terror" deliberately blurs the lines between crime, terrorism, and warfare. It melds nonstate terrorism with "preemptive war" doctrine. Domestic and international boundaries effectively vanish. Despite Posse Comitatis law limiting the military in domestic affairs to dealing with "rebellion," military jurisdiction expands into the domestic arena.[20] In turn, practices unique to counterterrorism, like "rendition" and the extraterritorial status of

Guantanamo, challenge both military and civil law and their respective traditions. In a further move toward isolation, an "intelligence czar" brings together agencies like the FBI, the CIA, the intelligence units of the respective military services, and about ten others that in one way or another deal with homeland security.[21] As George Annas reminds us, "draconian quarantine measures would probably have the unintended effect of encouraging people to avoid public health officials and physicians. . . . In this regard, the protection of civil liberties is a core ingredient in a successful response to a bioterrorist attack. Provisions that treat citizens as the enemy . . . are much more likely to cost lives than to save them."[22]

Ironically, terrorism is nourished rather than defeated by our practices and policies. Thus,

> A stark assessment of terrorism trends by American intelligence agencies has found that the American invasion and occupation of Iraq has helped spawn a new generation of Islamic radicalism. . . . The intelligence estimate, completed in April [2006], is the first formal appraisal of global terrorism by United States intelligence agencies since the Iraq war began, and represents a consensus view of the sixteen disparate spy services inside government. Titled "Trends in Global Terrorism: Implications for the United States," it asserts that Islamic radicalism, rather than being in retreat, has metastasized and spread across the globe. An opening section of the report, "Indicators of the Spread of the Global *Jihadist* Movement," cites the Iraq war as a reason for the diffusion of *jihad* ideology.[23]

The "war on terror" ranging from 9/11 to the Madrid bombings and from Saddam Hussein to Osama bin Laden is *sui generis*. It encourages domestic behaviors that are not typical of public health, clinical medicine, criminal justice, or the military tradition. With Iraq II conceived as part of the "war on terror," these institutions struggle to adapt to urban warfare, civil war, ideological motivation, and religious belief. Thus the confusion we witness about strategy and tactics, about secrecy, about executive power and its limits. Thus, too, questions of law and of ethics appear that are met with vague and dubious replies—for example, are terrorists prisoners of war; is indefinite imprisonment acceptable; are secret trials legitimate? Does justice distinguish between citizens and noncitizens?

Remembering Korea and Vietnam, the military does not want to be accused of fighting this "war" with the strategies of the last one. At the same time, it is unprepared to fight a "war" that isn't a war. An essay published by the Strategic Studies Institute of the U.S. Army notes,

> The administration has postulated a multiplicity of enemies, including rogue states; weapons of mass destruction proliferators; terrorist organizations of global, regional, and national scope; and terrorism itself. It also seems to have conflated them into a monolithic threat, and in so doing has subordinated stra-

> tegic clarity to the moral clarity it strives for in foreign policy and may have set the United States on a course of open-ended and gratuitous conflict with states and non-state entities that pose no serious threat to the United States. . . . If there is an analogy for the GWOT [global war on terrorism], it is the international war on illicit narcotics. But these "wars" on terrorism and drugs are not really wars as most Americans, including the professional military, have come to understand the meaning of the term since the United States became a world power.[24]

The Law of Nations

Memories of the first attack (1993) on the Twin Towers were very much alive for a while. For example, immediately after the Oklahoma bombing (1995), the search for perpetrators automatically looked to radical Islam. They turned out to be "homegrown." In the years after 9/11, plotters or suspected plotters, Muslim and homegrown as well, as in Buffalo and Los Angeles, got their headlines and their jail sentences. Thanks to the PATRIOT Acts, association itself became a crime. For example,

> An American citizen convicted of receiving training at a terrorist camp alongside members of Al Qaeda in his efforts to help overthrow the Somali government was sentenced to ten years in prison. The man, Daniel J. Maldonado, twenty-eight, a Muslim convert also known as Daniel Aljughaifi and Abu Mohammed, also received a $1,000 fine. Mr. Maldonado admitted to traveling in December to a terrorist camp in Somalia. Members of Al Qaeda were at the camp. Mr. Maldonado was captured in Kenya in January and brought back to the United States in February. He grew up in Pelham, N.H., but lived in Houston for four months in 2005 before moving with his wife and children to Cairo.[25]

Preventing an event, as in the "plot" to blow up fuel tanks at Kennedy Airport (2007), was a time for self-congratulation. As the Kennedy story emeiged, however, the four alleged plotters turned out to be the "gang that couldn't shoot straight." A former federal prosecutor commented, "There unfortunately has been a tendency to shout too loudly about such cases. . . . To the extent that you over-hype a case, you create fear and paranoia."[26] As if to verify his comment, an explosion in mid-town Manhattan (July 2007) quickly evoked memories of 9/11. Terrorism was an immediate reaction although, as quickly became evident, a broken steam pipe was the cause. In almost mythic fashion bin Laden has become an omnipresent villain and jihadism an omnipresent causal agent. Certainly he continues to be a visible presence. But, reality denies mythology.

> Bin Laden's days as the movement's guiding star are over. The United States' most formidable nemesis now is not the Saudi terrorist leader but his nominal deputy, Ayman al-Zawahiri. Part impresario, part visionary, bin Laden made himself and the terrorist organization he co-founded into household words. To-

> day they are paired global "brands" as recognizable and interchangeable as any leading corporation and its high-visibility CEO. But mounting evidence suggests that his time of active involvement in al-Qaeda operations is behind him. Forced into hiding, he has ceased to be a major force in al-Qaeda planning and decision-making and, even more astonishing, in its public relations activities.[27]

Yet, despite the familiar warning of "heightened" risk in the *National Intelligence Estimate*—the latest as I write was issued in July 2008—no terrorist event has taken place in the United States since 2001.

Terrorism is international, so counterterror must be international. Thus, the Office of the Director of National Intelligence reported,

> We assess that greatly increased worldwide counterterrorism efforts over the past five years have constrained the ability of al-Qa'ida to attack the US Homeland again and have led terrorist groups to perceive the Homeland as a harder target to strike than on 9/11. These measures have helped disrupt known plots against the United States since 9/11. We are concerned, however, that this level of international cooperation may wane as 9/11 becomes a more distant memory and perceptions of the threat diverge.[28]

Decades ago the UN set out to control bioterrorism. The story of what happened along the way illustrates the frustrating environment in which internationalism operates. Back then, we were in the midst of the Cold War. Nuclear weapons were spreading to Asia and the Middle East, and biochemical weapons threatened to follow. With near unanimity, the Biological Weapons Convention was completed in 1972. It banned the production, use, and stockpiling of "Bacteriological [biological] and Toxin Weapons" and called for the destruction of all existing supplies. There was precedent for it in the 1925 Geneva Protocol prohibiting the use of poison gas in warfare.

The Cold War is over, science and technology have become more accessible, and new players, "nonstate actors," have entered the international arena. A seeming success, by 2006, 155 states were "parties" to the Convention. But only sixteen states—primarily from the "third world"—became signatories. None of the major industrial nations including the United States have ratified the Convention (i.e., have given it the force of law). Perhaps illustrating a rule of sovereignty—the bugbear that haunts international endeavors—the higher the stakes, the more likely that nations will suspect their neighbors and insist on protecting themselves. Cynically, perhaps, the less likely to support effective law, the greater the increase of moralistic rhetoric.

The Convention called for a series of five-year reviews. At the 1980 session, it was interpreted to apply to "all international, national, and nonstate actors," thus bringing bioterrorism within its purview. The fifth review in 2001, however, was suspended "because of divergent positions" in the working committee. Reconvening a year later, the "states parties" agreed to several procedural changes; for example, to hold annual expert meetings, to "discuss and promote common understanding," and to encourage "national measures to implement the prohibitions set forth in the Convention." By 2006, the Convention was focused on a series of declarations whose language is laden with terms like "conviction, determination, reaffirmation." Finally, the parties "solemnly declare: their conviction that the Convention is essential for international peace and security."[29] If my skeptic's reading of international organization is accurate, this signals the end of meaningful law-making for the time being.

The Convention remains in place. However, U.S. policy and that of other nations is symptomatic.

> On the grounds of a military base . . . the Bush administration is building a massive biodefense laboratory unlike any seen since biological weapons were banned thirty-four years ago. . . . The work at this new lab, at Fort Detrick, Md., could someday save thousands of lives—or, some fear, create new risks and place the United States in violation of international treaties. . . . A computer slide show prepared by the center's directors in 2004 . . . suggests the lab will be making and testing small amounts of weaponized microbes and, perhaps, genetically engineered viruses and bacteria. . . . "If we saw others doing this kind of research, we would view it as an infringement of the bioweapons treaty," said Milton Leitenberg, a senior research scholar and weapons expert at the University of Maryland's School of Public Policy. . . . "All the programs we do are defensive in nature," said Maureen McCarthy, Homeland Security's director of research and development, who oversees NBACC [National Biodefense Analysis and Countermeasures Center].[30]

Of course, without weaponized microbes and engineered viruses, it is impossible to develop methods of prevention and treatment. Biology has its own ironies: the same knowledge and the same processes also make bioterror attack possible.

BLACK BOX

Bioterrorism will happen, will probably happen, is unlikely to happen, will not happen. Or we can conjugate "to know," as in we know we are being attacked, we will know we're being attacked, we may know we're being attacked, we may never know we've been attacked. In short, it is not possible to conclude very much with certainty.

As I've said, the terrorism of bombs and battles is theater, and terrorists need theater. The weakness of nonstate actors is masked by performance—costume, masks, pronouncements, media portrayals, and so on. Nations too, under certain circumstances, resort to theater and often for the same reasons. Thus, "shock and awe" in Iraq II supported a "lean and mean" and inadequate military force. The bombing of Nagasaki and Hiroshima demonstrated nuclear weaponry, but these were only two bombs available. The shouts and bugles of Chinese troops announced mass infantry attacks in the Korean War.

Bioterror, by contrast, is a quiet weapon. To be sure, all terrorism deals in threat and anxiety; but bioterrorism perfects them. It conquers no territories, brings down no planes, destroys no armaments. And it doesn't have to. It is a psychological and cultural weapon as much as a biological one. And it appeals to memory and history. It evokes the images and smells and not just the casualties of plague and pox, the pictures of rats and mosquitoes and fleas invading the body's private spaces, the sight of child or parent or husband or wife, wasting away while others stand by helpless, the corruption of food and water that beyond nourishment stands for home and community. Bioterror, in other words, counters our resort to rationality, i.e., to the technology of war. While relying on modern science, bioterrorism plays to the most irrational features of our being. The headlines and fear-mongering out of all proportion to events are understandable. We react!

The necessary but not the sufficient condition of bioterror is scientific development or better, news of scientific development. In the absence of attack, it makes bioterror believable, the threat believable. Looking forward, David Relman, a former editor of the *New England Journal of Medicine*, wrote,

> How well founded is this heightened concern about bioterrorism? . . . [W]e cannot assume that the logic behind bio-warfare programs of the past will guide future misuses of the life sciences. Indeed, the lessons of this history can be dangerously misleading. First, the notion that only a certain few agents pose a plausible threat is largely an artifact of weapons programs that predated our current knowledge of molecular biology. . . Furthermore, large-scale industrial processes are not necessary for the development of potent biologic weapons. . . . Even our traditional concept of "weaponization" is misleading: nature provides mechanisms for packaging and preserving many infectious agents that can be manipulated through biologic and genetic engineering. . . . Materials science and nanoscale science—advances in encapsulation technology, for instance—will provide new ways to package such agents. And self-replicating agents that are highly transmissible among humans, such as variola virus and influenza virus, need little or no alteration in order to be disseminated efficiently by terrorists.[31]

If Relman is correct, then the biology and technology of bioterror will improve and will be widely accessible. And, if terrorism matures, moving beyond the primitive methodology of bombs and battles, then bioterrorism may well become a weapon of choice. That will call for preparing to meet the usual problems—sudden attacks and mass casualties—with both standard and novel responses. It will also generate new pressures for security and censorship.[32] Along the way, without intending it, terror and counterterror become even more like mirror images of each other, resorting to similar weapons and practices. But counterterror is just that, reactive. The terrorist enjoys the advantage of a first strike. Each side, of course, claims its virtue, the moral reasons for its action.

Responding to bioterrorism with counterterrorism, e.g., weaponizing bacteria, enforcing security, closing off financial resources, leaves the *threat* of bioterror untouched. Threats, after all, can neither be captured nor assassinated. In short, counterterror calls for a cultural strategy in order to achieve a society that can absorb bioterrorism (i.e., absorb the threat) and still maintain its democratic integrity.

Such a strategy would need to generate communitywide scientific literacy. The public and not just the expert would understand that probability is knowledge at its best. Historically, with the move to sciences that rely on evidence, statistical methods, and continued self-criticism, we also moved to sciences that stir the imagination and create useable and fascinating ideas and technologies. Uncertainty, in other words, is creative. Absorbing this lesson, the "quest for certainty" becomes not merely a metaphysical error and psychological stumbling block but irrelevant. As it were, a scientific culture would "outgrow" it.

For most of us, however, the sciences are a black box. We appropriate the results of technology without understanding or appreciating how they came to be and how they work. We excuse our ignorance by referring science to scientists and denying the need to do much more than that. We also deny that we are capable of understanding what is going on. Science, mathematics, and engineering are not the most popular major studies in our universities. Secondary school instruction is more often than not amateurish and outdated. But, few complain or even understand that a complaint is justified. It need not be that way. When interest or passion stir our curiosity, we probe and learn, and do. In short, we demonstrate that we can be competent. We also live successfully with uncertainties on our jobs and in our recreations. We deal with the odds in our romance with sports and gambling, with the results of polls and surveys. Isolating terrorism behind the walls of counterterrorism, both a reflection of our cultural habits and a reinforcement of them, defeats these capacities. In the "war on terror" we become clients and victims. We are encouraged to be passive, which is by no means the same as a considered decision to *do* nothing.

A cultural strategy would aim to dissolve the aura of threat and anxiety that is terrorism's strength. But it would not be an easy strategy. As Albert Einstein half a century ago wrote, "It is, in fact, nothing short of a miracle that the modern methods of instruction have not yet entirely strangled the holy curiosity of inquiry."[33] Good science and mathematics teaching are still in short supply and the media, by and large, reinforce the black box that is our image of the sciences. A cultural strategy would challenge political and economic interests that are served by keeping things as they are. The mirror image would be shattered.

But things are not that simple. We are ephemeral creatures who are born, live, and die, creatures always with a sense of insecurity lurking in shadows of consciousness. So, existential anxiety will not entirely vanish even if counterterrorism learns the lessons of a democratic society. The appeal of certainty will remain. The cultural lesson must be taught over and over again.

NOTES

1. "Existentialism," *Stanford Encyclopedia of Philosophy*, 2004.

2. "New World Coming: American Security in the 21st Century, Major Themes and Implications." The Phase I Report on the Emerging Global Security Environment for the First Quarter of the 21st Century, The United States Commission on National Security/21st Century, September 15, 1999, Gary Hart and Warren Rudman, Chairs.

3. Hans Vaihinger, a Kant scholar, published his *Philosophie des Als Ob* (*Philosophy of As If*) in 1911. He argued that we can never really know the underlying reality of the world. Consequently, we construct systems of thought and then behave "as-if" the world matches them. Unlike metaphysical determinism, however, "as if" includes methods of criticism and validation. For example, protons, electrons, and electromagnetic waves are not directly observed. However, using indirect observations to "verify" or "falsify" their "existence," physicists modify existing theoretical constructs or create new ones.

4. In the previous chapter, we cited Dark Winter. Blue Advance–02 assumed a smallpox attack on Puerto Rico. In the evaluation, the move from assumption to actual policy recommendations is obvious. See, "Smallpox Strikes Puerto Rico in Bioterrorism Exercise, Lessons Learned from Exercise Blue Advance-02," Joint Center for Lessons Learned, March 2004.

5. "Is There Still a Terrorist Threat?" John Mueller, *Foreign Affairs*, September/October 2006. On-line summary at http://www.foreignaffairs.org/20060901facomment85501/john-mueller/is-there-still-a-terrorist-threat.html3.

6. "Is There Still a Terrorist Threat?"

7.

> There are several reasons why the vulnerability of U.S. agriculture might not be appreciated. A recent RAND study notes, "Most Americans take it for granted that food is readily available and that their food is safe." A second reason that agriculture is "invisible" is that "modern agricultural practices in the United States, which are increasingly concentrated, have led to a dramatic reduction in the number of farms (2.2 million in 1998 compared to 6.3 million in 1929)." A third reason is that "technological innovation has resulted in

fewer Americans being directly employed in agricultural production: farming accounted for 2 percent of the U.S. workforce in 1998 down from 23 percent in 1929." The vertical integration of agribusinesses—that is, the concentration of activities related to food production and distribution—also contributes to their susceptibility to attack.

"Agroterrorism in the U.S.: Key Security Challenges for the 21st Century," O. Shawn Cupp, David E. Walker II, and John Hillison, *Biosecurity and Bioterrorism: Biodefense Strategy, Practice, and Science,* Volume 2, Number 2, 2004, p. 98.

8. "The Precautionary Principle," Peter Montague, *Rachel's Environment and Health Weekly* #586, 2/19/05.

9. See: "Heralding Unheard Voices: The Role of Faith-Based Organizations and Nongovernmental Organizations during Disasters," Final Report, Science and Technology Directorate, Department of Homeland Security, December 2006.

10. "Bioterrorism Preparedness, Cooptation of Public Health?" Victor W. Sidel, MD; Robert M. Gould, MD; Hillel W. Cohen, PhD, *Medicine & Global Survival,* Vol. 7, No. 2, February 2002, p. 85.

11. "Biocrimes, Microbial Forensics, and the Physician," Steven E. Schutzer, Bruce Budowle, Ronald M. Atlas, Public Forum, *PLoS Med* 2(12): e337, 09/27/05.

12. See "Bioterrorism and the People: How to Vaccinate a City against Panic," Thomas A. Glass and Monica Schoch-Spana, *Clinical Infectious Diseases,* 34, 01/15/02, pp. 217–23.

13. "The London Attacks—Response," a series of articles in the *NEJM,* Volume 353, 6, 08/11/05.

14. "Policing Terrorism," David Rieff, *NYT,* 7/21/07.

15.

Acting more quickly than in 2001 when chaos gripped the farming industry, the government imposed an immediate nationwide ban on the movement of cattle, pigs and sheep. . . . Agricultural officials from the Department for Environment, Food and Rural Affairs donned white overalls and swarmed over the summer green rural region in Surrey. . . . There was some confidence that the quicker measures would help stave off the devastating spread of the disease in 2001 when more than four million animals were slaughtered and many farmers were put out of business. . . . Tourism fell sharply, too, in 2001. Today, government officials were at pains to say that the British countryside, now clogged with local and foreign vacationers, was open for unrestricted travel. In 2001, many trails, forests and national parkland were kept off limits after the outbreak.

"Britain Responds to Foot-and-Mouth Outbreak," Jane Perlez, *NYT,* 8/4/07.

16.

Collaboration with law enforcement officials generally has not been recognized as beneficial or desirable in public health. The presence of law enforcement officers has been thought to compromise the collection of sensitive medical information (e.g., illegal drug use). . . . Law enforcement is now increasingly focused on prevention of terrorist acts, requiring a new partnership with the public health and medical community. The steps necessary to identify a potential covert bioterrorism attack include a close coordination between those who collect and analyze medical and syndromic surveillance information with the law-enforcement community's intelligence and case-related information. The best method for timely detection of a covert bioterrorist attack is early communication between the two communities and recognition of the extent and origin of the threat.

"Collaboration between Public Health and Law Enforcement: New Paradigms and Partnerships for Bioterrorism Planning and Response," Jay C. Butler, Mitchell L. Cohen, Cindy R. Friedman, Robert M. Scripp, and Craig G. Watz, *Emerging Infectious Diseases*, Vol. 8, No. 10, October 2002, pp. 1152–56.

17. The major international exception was former British Prime Minister, Tony Blair, who shared with President Bush the rhetoric of a "war on terror." In practice, however, the British continued to treat terrorism as a criminal matter.

18. "2 British Antiterror Experts Say U.S. Takes Wrong Path," Raymond Bonner, *NYT*, 10/22/08.

19. "Overview of America's National Strategy for Combating Terrorism," White House, *NSC*, 9/5/06.

20.

> Whenever the President considers that unlawful obstructions, combinations, or assemblages, or rebellion against the authority of the United States, make it impracticable to enforce the laws of the United States in any State or Territory by the ordinary course of judicial proceedings, he may call into Federal service such of the militia of any State, and use such of the armed forces, as he considers necessary to enforce those laws or to suppress the rebellion.

"Military Power in Law Enforcement: The Posse Comitatus," United States Constitution, Article II, Constitutional Law Center, annotation.

21. See, *NCTC [National Counterterrorism Center] and Information Sharing: Five Years since 9/11: A Progress Report, 9/06*. NCTC hosts a classified repository, NCTC Online (NOL), that serves as the counterterrorism community's library of terrorism information. This repository reaches the full range of intelligence, law enforcement, military, homeland security, and other federal organizations involved in the global war on terrorism. The creation of NOL, coupled with policy changes, has allowed nonintelligence community agencies easier access to counterterrorism information and has resulted in broad and robust sharing of intelligence information. Today, NOL hosts over 6,000 users, 6 million documents, over 60 contributing departments and agencies.

22. *Bioterrorism, Public Health, and Civil Liberties*, George J. Annas, J.D., M.P.H., *NEJM*, Volume 346, No. 17, 4/25/02, pp. 1337–42.

23. "Spy Agencies Say Iraq War Worsens Terror Threat," Mark Mazzetti, *NYT*, 9/24/06.

24. "Bounding the Global War on Terrorism," Jeffrey Record, *Strategic Studies Institute* [SSI], U.S. Army War College, Carlisle, PA, December 2003.

25. "Texas: Sentence in Terrorism Training," *Associated Press*, 7/22/07.

26. "Experts Cast Doubt on Credibility of JFK Terror Plot," Luis Torres de la Llosa, *Agence France Presse*, 6/5/07.

27. "Scarier Than Bin Laden," Bruce Hoffman, *Washington Post*, 9/9/07.

28. "The Terrorist Threat to the U.S. Homeland," National Intelligence Estimate, July 2007.

29. These comments are based on "Sixth Review Conference of the States Parties to the Biological Weapons Convention," November 2006, Geneva.

30. "The Secretive Fight Against Bioterror," (The government is building a highly classified facility to research biological weapons, but its closed-door approach has raised concerns.) Joby Warrick, *Washington Post*, 7/30/06.

31. "Bioterrorism—Preparing to Fight the Next War," David A. Relman, MD, *NEJM*, Volume 354, 2, 01/12/06, p. 113.

32. For a discussion of some of the issues involved in the censorship of scientific information, see, "A Tale of Two Studies: Ethics, Bioterrorism, and the Censorship of Science," Michael J. Selgelid, Hastings Center Report 37, no. 3, 2007, pp. 35–43.

33. "Autobiographical Notes," *Albert Einstein: Philosopher-Scientist*, The Library of Living Philosophers, Paul Arthur Schilpp, editor, Evanston, Illinois, 1949, p. 17.

10

Conclusions and Confusions

TERROR AND TERRORISM

Katrina, SARS, flu, pox, and anthrax illustrate the characteristics of catastrophe. Of course, other events could have been chosen; for example, the Southeast Asia tsunami, Three-Mile Island, the London bombings, and so on. Each is unique as all events are unique. And yet, each affects how we feel, how we think, how we see ourselves, how we see each other, and how we see the world. Each intensifies our feelings of vulnerability. Finally, each teaches the lessons of terror.

> As captured in the Greek roots of the words "catastrophe" and "cataclysm," a disaster is a violent overthrowing of the status quo—an event that dramatically ruptures everyday expectations about physical survival, the social order, and the meaning of life . . . Watershed events like disasters and epidemics provoke political after-effects, transform social expectations and institutions, and create indelible personal memories. . . . Galveston, Texas, which was successfully rebuilt after the 1900 storm that killed 8,000 and washed three-quarters of the town away, never recovered its prominence as one of the nation's wealthiest communities, and it was soon eclipsed by Houston, the state's oil hub and emerging port city. Hurricane Katrina created the largest internal diaspora of Americans since the Civil War, prompted rancorous government hearings and restructuring measures, and left viewers across the country and the world with lasting and graphic video images of human suffering.[1]

Floods, hurricanes, and earthquakes make us victims. We struggle against them; we prepare and mobilize; we explain and interpret. We try to retake control of our lives, thus proving that we are not helpless as victims are helpless in the midst of chaos. Failing that, which is almost inevitable, we try to give catastrophe meaning, try to make it intelligible. But ultimately, catastrophe just happens.

In the event, we help and are helped by the stranger, now made familiar by a shared destiny.

> How the disaster starts does not matter: It could be a plane crashing into the World Trade Center, it could be the sea receding rapidly ahead of an advancing tsunami, it could be smoke billowing through a nightclub. . . . Human beings in New York, Sri Lanka and Rhode Island all do the same thing in such situations. They turn to each other. They talk. They hang around, trying to arrive at a shared understanding of what is happening. . . . Contrary to the notion of selfish behavior in crises . . . the accounts of how people fled the World Trade Center building on Sept. 11 reveal only one instance of a man who heard an explosion, laced up his tennis shoes and ran until he was far away from the building.[2]

In our time, terrorism, no longer a sometime military tactic or the finite intrusion of personal violence into public life, pervades our consciousness. The terrors of experience are reinforced by terrorism. We divide humanity into friends and enemies. We look warily at each other—whose side are you on? We search out villainy or invent it. We have become targets. The stranger alters once again, becoming ambiguously both familiar and threatening. Terrorism thus invites anger and hate to the table, signaling its difference from the fears of "normal" terror. Authority becomes ambiguous, too. The caregiver becomes the policeman; the policeman becomes the soldier; the soldier becomes the counterterrorist. We all are changed.

In the event, natural or man-made, the obvious things get done. The dead are collected and disposed of. The wounded are treated. The frightened are comforted. The imperatives of public health and clinical medicine guide our acts. No longer just victims, we are cared for and not just done to. But, with terrorism, less obvious things also are done. Evidence is gathered. The search for causes—of infection, of flooded neighborhoods, of collapsed buildings—is reconfigured by purpose. Someone, after all, intends our pain and our destruction.

A "war on terrorism" prolongs our anonymity.

> In wartime, language must be created to enable combatants and noncombatants alike to see the other side as killable, to overcome the innate queasiness over the taking of human life. Soldiers, and those who remain at home, learn to call their enemies by names that make them seem not quite human—inferior, contemptible and not like "us." . . . So some terms of war are collective nouns, encouraging us to see the enemy as an undifferentiated mass, rather than as individuals capable of suffering. Crusaders called their enemy "the Saracen," and in World War I, the British called Germans "the Hun." American

soldiers are trained to call those they are fighting against "the enemy." It is easier to kill an enemy than an Iraqi.[3]

We become objects. No longer owning personal names and histories, we acquire an attributed collective identity. We become the enemy's enemy—variously, these days, unbelievers, invaders, exploiters. Our fear, pain, and death are a tactic, a means of communication, political and ideological, to the other as enemy. The claim of innocence, as in "innocent bystander," is dismissed. There are no innocents! We become instrumental to ends not our own.

Nature terrorizes without purpose. The waters, the heavens, the trembling earth, have no intention, no personality, no viewpoint. To be sure, it will have partners—error or incompetence or negligence as we have seen. But these are lesser partners of the larger phenomenon. We resent being incidental outcomes of a natural event—the "absurd" as my existentialist friends used to say. We may feel—we want to feel—that we have been done to and that it—some it—has done it to us. Hence, the myths, sacred and secular, that we invent to personalize causality give it reasons and ourselves excuses.

Ironically, terrorism is easier. There is an enemy, a purpose, an agent. But other puzzles less manageable appear. Not who I am but where and when I am makes me the enemy's enemy. The bullet or rocket that kills me is indifferent kin to the bullet or rocket that kills the enemy. For terrorism, why and where I am—the attributed "I" again—not who I am is relevant, perhaps the most relevant thing about me. I kill for a reason. I am killed for a reason. And yet, the reasons on all sides remain abstract, collective, even where the passions they stir are not.

FROM ARISTOTLE TO MARX

With the rhetoric of a "war" on terrorism comes a moral puzzle: there seems to be no reliable way of distinguishing between virtue and villainy. Accident of birth or place is as likely as not to announce their difference. Virtue and vice are thus rooted in the arbitrary. Dependent on position and situation, ethics is reduced to custom and locality. It may have its reasons—survival perhaps, self-interest perhaps, social solidarity perhaps—but it remains a species of self-justification. Patriotism and propaganda convince me of my virtue. But the other too is convinced, is also a patriot. Even at the extremes of life and death, moral illusion rules. For example,

> Just exactly what distinguishes the United States' use of the ever-so-cutely-named "Fat Man" and "Little Boy" atomic bombs on cities in Japan from the car bombs of Baghdad or the planes that smashed into the World Trade Center? . . . Of

course, we had our justifications, as terrorists always do. Truman defended his decision to drop the atomic bombs on civilians over the objection of leading atomic scientists on the grounds that it was a necessary military action to save lives by forcing a quick Japanese surrender. . . . The subsequent release of formerly secret documents makes a hash of Truman's rationalization. His White House was fully informed that the Japanese were on the verge of collapse, and their surrender was made all the more likely by the Soviets' imminent entry into the fight.[4]

Three things follow, none of them very neat. The first is a caution against the moral absolutism of warfare. Invited to righteousness, I allocate virtue to me and mine and vice to the other. I am thus authorized to destroy and kill and to explain away as "collateral damage" the "innocents," not really innocent, caught in the web of battle. Thus,

> Critics have rightly pointed out that traditional categories of combatant and civilian are muddled in a struggle against terrorists. In a traditional war, combatants and civilians are relatively easy to distinguish. The 9/11 hijackers, by contrast, dressed in ordinary clothes and hid their weapons. They acted not as citizens of Saudi Arabia, an ally of America, but as members of Al Qaeda, a shadowy transnational network. And their prime targets were innocent civilians. By treating such terrorists as combatants, however, we accord them a mark of respect and dignify their acts. And we undercut our own efforts against them in the process. . . . Labeling its members as combatants elevates its cause and gives *Al Qaeda* an undeserved status.[5]

When terrorism is understood as crime, the moral opportunism of warfare is dissolved. Law and tradition—national and international law, military and civil law—serve a moral end. Ultimately an appeal to justice enables a line between virtue and vice. We can judge, condemn, and punish. We acquire the opportunity—for example, declarations and treaties on human rights, international conventions—to cross the boundaries between "us" and "them." To be sure, laws are imperfect moral instruments. But they are familiar as the criminal is familiar. Of course, that has its moral risk, too. We are tempted to alienate the other in a different way, as in, "To understand all is to forgive all." All unaware, we claim moral superiority. Ethics is all too easily transformed into sentimentality and self-congratulation.

Second is a reminder. In war, there are aggressors and defenders. But, distinguishing between the two is not as easy as we sometimes think. To be sure, exploding the first bomb is, *prima facie,* an act of aggression. Bombing the bomber is, *prima facie,* an act of defense. But, what are we to make of "preemptive" strikes or of providing terrorists with financial aid? It is difficult enough to divide aggressor and defender in traditional warfare where a "declaration of war" is explicit and where invasion or attack announces the shift from negotiation to destruction. "War is diplomacy carried on by other means," wrote Von Clausewitz, not cynically but descriptively. All too often, however, it is the victor who in the end names aggressor and defender. A commentator, for example, attempts to escape the dubious ethical status of "preemption" by distinguishing it from "prevention." But, once again, as with so much of the language of warfare, this distinction is a privilege of the strong and not the weak.

Third, terrorism is a weapon of last resort, a weapon of desperation. It is experienced by its targets as irrational, even self-defeating. But terrorism has its reasons—its plot line to recall terror's theatricality—that explain but do not necessarily excuse. It has its history too, but calling it "history" already betrays our cultural location, Western and secular. For Hindu, Buddhist, or Taoist, history is surrendered to the endlessness of time, eternal recurrence, the dissolution of our world of appearance, and the rhythmic tension between yin and yang. For the children of Abraham, drama replaces history; or better, history is drama, fitting events together in a grand epic of damnation and redemption. In short, the history of history does not flow neatly.

Ambiguity and contradiction are thus the "back story" of bioethics in a time of terrorism. There is no reliable way to avoid being situated. Western again, the Platonist in each of us thankfully seeks the good, the true, and the beautiful in the "heaven beyond the heavens." There is something satisfying to us in freeing the ideal from the grubbiness of the world. No less grand but less pleasing aesthetically, Kant's "pure practical reason" continues to celebrate our love affair with rationality. And, like many love affairs, things become all the more bitter as reason stumbles before events. The Western story is not, however, univocal. Early on, Aristotle reminded Plato that reason's ethics is shaped by political and psychological realities. And Karl Marx, still a child of the Enlightenment, reminded us that in a market-enchanted culture, power and status frame the moral questions we ask and the moral answers we give. Thus it is that terrorism, like all extreme conditions, forces us to leave the comforts of the "marketplace of ideas" and enter the marketplace of conduct and feeling. The moral environment is always the complicated and contradictory world of human events and relationships. In a time of terrorism, it becomes even more complicated and contradictory.

DEMOCRATIC DILEMMAS

Western thought has treated moral ideas as universal although the pluralities of today's world subvert the notion.[6] Are we then trapped in moral anarchy? Ethics is formed in particular ways and within particular perspectives. If not the majesty of universals, commonalities appear once we invoke the term *democracy*, as many now do globally or once we seek a utilitarian's calculus. Participation and discourse are indeed constitutive democratic values. But cultural comparisons show that they are rooted in human beings as such, are necessities in dealing effectively with human affairs just about anywhere.

Catastrophe makes the point clear when it opts for a command society in the name of efficiency. A command society does not worry about representation and transparency and the like, nor does it regard their absence as morally problematic. At the same time, such a society deals poorly with the catastrophic; that is, experiencing greater numbers of casualties, taking longer to recover, and so on. Duty, in a command society, appears as absolute obedience to the state or to the leader. Yet duty, without intimacy, quickly becomes going through the motions. "I was only obeying orders," reveals duty's mechanization. Autonomy—self-governance—is replaced by the demands of the superior on the inferior. The alienation of leader and follower built into a command society sooner or later creates problems of practice; for example, loss of initiative and shared intelligence, avoidance of duties unless under direct observation, excuse-giving in the presence of failure, and so on. A command society deliberately rejects the transactional dimensions of human being, a notion captured by the fact that we are social and political animals. Thus, it lacks the strengths of participation. To be sure, the moral issues that arise for us might not arise under different social and political conditions. The consequences that would trouble the democrat might not trouble the commander. Yet, these brief remarks—emerging from our look at SARS and flu for example—tell us that situatedness is not relativism, i.e., not all situations are created equal. In the moral situation, reality, sooner or later, will call the tune for democrat and autocrat alike.

A striking illustration of the "situatedness" of bioethics appears in the military's reconstruction of its role in a time of terrorism. The newly issued *Counterinsurgency Manual* includes three sections that are particularly relevant.[7] Thus, the section on "Ethics" includes the following:

> One of the insurgents' most effective means to undermine and erode political will is to portray their opposition as untrustworthy or illegitimate. These attacks are especially effective when insurgents can portray the opposition as unethical by their own standards. To combat these efforts, Soldiers and Marines treat noncombatants and detainees humanely and in accordance with America's values and internationally recognized human rights standards. In COIN [counter-insurgency], preserving noncombatant lives and dignity is central to mission accomplishment. This imperative creates a complex ethical environment that requires combatants to treat prohibitions against harming noncombatants as absolute. Further, it can sometimes require combatants to forego lethal solutions altogether. In practical terms, this consideration means that mission accomplishment sometimes obligates combatants to act more like police than warriors.[8]

No doubt responsive to Abu Ghraib and Guantanamo, the opening lines of the section on "Limits on Interrogation" read,

> Abuse of detained persons is immoral, illegal, and unprofessional. Those who engage in cruel or inhuman treatment of prisoners betray the standards of the profession of arms and the laws of the United States. . . . Torture and cruel, inhumane, and degrading treatment is never a morally permissible option, even in situations where lives depend on gaining information. No exceptional circumstances permit the use of torture and other cruel, inhuman or degrading treatment.[9]

To drive home its views, the *Manual* cites French conduct in Algeria. The vignette is entitled, "Lose Moral Legitimacy, Lose the War."

> During Algerian war of independence between 1954 and 1962, French leaders decided to permit torture against suspected insurgents. Though they were aware that it was against the law and morality of war, they argued that (1) this was a new form of war and these rules did not apply; (2) the threat the enemy represented, communism, was a great evil that justified extraordinary means; and (3) the application of torture against insurgents was measured and nongratuitous. This official condoning of torture . . . empowered the moral legitimacy of the opposition, undermined the French moral legitimacy, and caused internal fragmentation among serving officers that led to an unsuccessful coup attempt in 1962. In the end, failure to comply with moral and legal restrictions against torture severely undermined French efforts and contributed to their loss despite a number of significant military victories. Illegal and immoral activities made the counterinsurgents extremely vulnerable to enemy propaganda inside Algeria among the Muslim population, as well as in the United Nations and the French media. These actions also degraded the ethical climate throughout the French Army. France eventually recognized Algerian independence in July, 1963.[10]

It would not do to ignore "moral luck," as Bernard Williams put it, or *fortuna,* as Machiavelli put it. But both terrorism and counterterrorism do. Both attempt the grandiose, seeing themselves as world forming and as world reforming. Thus, the effort to convert the world too any single belief system like Islam or Christianity or communism, or to any univocal norm like a market economy. The ideological move forecasts failure.[11] The world does not yield to our wishes or to our fears. It is surely not finally controlled by us.

In order to make moral sense, we cannot ignore the world's constraints. "Ought implies can" as the ethicist puts it. Commonalities are, in other words, ragged around the edges. We live in specific times and places, have specific biographies, enjoy specific hopes and dreams, are shaken by specific fears and threats. We face choices, have preferences. Nor is it surprising that the move from terror to terrorism has had its effects on how we identify and understand the moral issues we face and how we deal with them. Thus, democratic formalism persists; democratic substance is surrendered. With that, both conscience and credibility are put in jeopardy.

TRUST

Even under "normal" conditions, democratic values are challenged by catastrophe. With triage, our lives will be differently valued. Consent will surrender to exigency. Religious beliefs will be ignored or violated. Fairness will be put into question. In a time of terrorism, suspicion of emergency responses, already present, intensifies. Reason-giving becomes a security issue. Directives appear arbitrary and even mysterious. Explanations give way to orders. Secrecy, even justifiable secrecy, invites the corruption of information. In short, trust, already put at risk by the demands of "normal" catastrophe, becomes even more dubious.

To trust another or to be trusted by another signals our ability to deliberate, to communicate, and to act dependably. Trust, in other words, evokes a cluster of moral characteristics; for example, honor, truthfulness, reliability. When we trust, we recognize the humanity in each other. When we trust a government, a school, a church, we recognize the humanity of those who formulated their principles and practices and shaped their traditions and those who sustain them in the present. Even those institutions, like public corporations that celebrate the objectivity of their decisions and practices, reveal in their celebration that particular human minds and hands are at work. Else, such institutions would be carbon copies, clones of each other, and they are not. An institution, in other words, is a reflection of the humanity it embodies. In turn, its members are a reflection of the institutions of which they are a part.

Promise keeping is trust in action, a paradigmatic instance of trust. In making a promise, I announce that I expect to be trusted. When I keep a promise, I verify that expectation. If I fail to keep a promise I am obligated to explain why, to give good reasons for my failure. I also am obligated to discover any harms my failure has caused and to make restitution in some significant way. Institutions like governments and gods make and break promises, too. But beyond the facticity of a promise is its larger statement. A promise affirms the future when the promise is to be fulfilled and reaffirms the past that justifies us in believing each other when we invoke the future. Behind the promise is a metaphysical assertion; faith in the reliability of the world.

Of course, trust can be betrayed. Ordinarily, however, betrayal does not bring with it an environment of betrayal. Governments break promises all the time. But we turn to government itself for the remedy. It remains its own corrective even in so cynical a moment as our own. Similarly, in dealing with the scandal of an untrustworthy priesthood, it was the church in which the scandal was born to which believers turned for reform. In other words, trust can be affirmed in the very act of its violation. The possibility of remedy verifies the act of promising. Catastrophic events are moments when trust is at greatest risk. It is not incidental the rule of the sniper and the street gang in Katrina, for instance, followed a radical failure to perform on a promise; the covenant between governor and governed is broken. Terrorism, in this regard, is an index of the failure of promises and the failure of remedies. Counterterror then is not only a matter of weaponry and tactics but also of moral strategies.

TERRORISM AND COUNTERTERRORISM

With terrorism, trust becomes problematic. The methods of terrorism—sneak attacks, anonymous actors, promiscuous targets—exploit hiddenness. Terrorists melt into the population from which they came. My neighbor, indeed anyone, may be my destroyer. For example, the leadership of doctors and nurses—of "caregivers"—in the London and Glasgow bombing attempts surprised and shocked their fellow professionals. Yet, as Simon Wessely pointed out,

> The chair of the *British International Doctors' Association* called the involvement of doctors "beyond belief." But is it? Walter Laqueur, perhaps the foremost scholar of the darkest crimes of the 20th century and the rise of terrorism, first observed that doctors were disproportionately represented among the ranks of terrorists. George Habash, the founder of the *Popular Front for the Liberation of Palestine* and the man behind the aircraft hijackings of *Black September*, was a doctor. Mohammed al-Hindi received his medical degree in Cairo in 1980, returning to his native Gaza the following year to form *Islamic Jihad*. Ayman al-Zawahiri, Al Qaeda's number-two leader and "spokesman," is a surgeon. . . . Many doctors are driven by a sense of altruism to work in refugee camps, war zones, and disaster areas . . . But one can be motivated by a similar sense of idealism to wish not only to heal the individual patient but also to right the injustices that have produced the sickness, wounds, and death. The line has been crossed when the desire to change the world for the better becomes detached from any consideration of the consequences of one's actions.[12]

In a time of terrorism, just about anything or anyone can explode—or at least that is how it feels. The persistent threat of attack, even in the absence of the attack itself, shapes an environment of distrust. The shock of the familiar becoming unfamiliar corroborates that distrust.

Terrorism exhibits an age-old moral problem, the disconnect between ends and means. With that, terrorism reveals its essential immorality. Its ideal, and terrorists are idealists, is surrendered to weakness. This deadly marriage of weakness and idealism allows the use of any method that works or seems to work toward reaching the ideal ends in view. Sooner or later, however, this disconnect discredits the ideal itself. It is tainted by the opportunism of its anarchic methodology. At the deepest levels of belief and commitment, trust vanishes. Chaos begins as terrorism's method and ends as its master.

Counterterrorism becomes, as I have said, the mirror of its adversary. Language moves from communication to manipulation. Authority is exercised in secret, giving security or fear of panic as its reason. Challenged, it offers the paternalist excuse: that it knows best. Its acts—of assassination, of torture, of lie-telling—are done in the name of the good. At the same time, its agents are made immune both to law and conscience, a privilege of initiates of an elite society that refers to itself as the "intelligence community." Counterterror, in other words, is an inversion of moral society. Challenged, it claims the protection of necessity; "unfortunate but necessary" is the familiar phrase. Terrorism, we are told, forces our acts upon us. Finally, we learn another lesson that terrorism teaches. We become untrustworthy too, disconnecting means and ends. Trust becomes a moral illusion.

A DUTY TO CARE

Like trust, a duty to care is a moral requirement for effective response to the catastrophic. Yet, it has been reshaped, and not for the better, by the modern experience. Thucydides and Cicero, Athens and Rome, invoked the duty of the citizen. For the philosopher, doing one's duty was a moral good; failing to do one's duty, a moral evil. But that is mere formalism. In the world, duties attach to actual roles and positions, "My Station and Its Duties," as the nineteenth century idealist philosopher, F. H. Bradley, put it. In an industrial and urban society, however, we inhabit many "stations." We play many roles simultaneously. Conflicting duties are thus unavoidable. Despite the simplicity of the imperative, "Do your duty," it is not unusual to ask, "What is my duty?"

Duties may be commanded by reason, as with Kant. Or, they may require doing the "will of god" or of "the commander-in-chief" or of "the party." Duty entails both an agent and a recipient. I do my duty to a friend, a spouse, a child. I have a duty to myself, although that is better understood as integrity. Duty's object may be collective; that is, duty to the community, the state, or the church. And finally, duty's object may be ideal; that is, an ideology, a belief system, a cause. Duty has a public face—say by taking an oath, wearing a particular costume. At the same time, it is intimate, as conscience is intimate.

I may do my duty and yet do harm, as when in Melville's novella, it becomes Captain Vere's duty to hang Billy Budd for striking an officer who falsely accused him of planning mutiny.[13] For Kant, doing one's duty for duty's sake is a moral imperative. For Josiah Royce, duty entails loyalty and ultimately, "loyalty to loyalty." Alternatively, duty may be part of an exchange of duties as in a "social contract." Thus, Hobbes releases the subject from duties to the sovereign when the latter fails to do his duty; that is, by failing to keep the peace the king reveals that he is no longer sovereign. Duty is connected to competence. By accepting a role, I claim the ability to perform my duty.

Duty is coercive. When I am treated as an autonomous being, that coercion is self-imposed. When I must do another's will—do another's duty as if it were mine—I am a tool, not a person. But I am a person! At that point, my duty is rebellion—the ultimate available existential act of saying, "No."

For the caregiver, a "duty to care" is in its origin a sacred trust, a "calling." With the emergence of modern societies, however, we secularize roles and duties. Calling becomes profession. Yet, we still refer to "rights and privileges" on ceremonial occasions, thus connecting the professional back to the tradition. For example, a familiar form of the Hippocratic Oath reads in part,

> I swear by Apollo the physician and Aesclaepius . . . and all the gods and goddesses, that, according to my ability and judgment, I will keep this Oath. . . . Whatever houses I may visit, I will come for the benefit of the sick, remaining free of all intentional injustice, of all mischief and in particular of sexual relations with both female and male persons, be they free or slaves.[14]

These days just about any occupation, career or trade, is called a "profession." However, a "duty to care" echoes the historic professions of law, medicine, the military, teaching, and the clergy. These make a self-transcending demand; for example, acceptance of risk even of one's life, sacrifice of personal interest for the sake of another's need, and so on. In principle, therefore, professional acts can be neither bought nor sold.

A profession is knowledge-rich. This creates an essential inequality between the professional and those served by him or her. Consequently, a professional's duty is necessarily "fiduciary"; that is, he or she acts on behalf of another who in turn entrusts the professional with what are vital interests—health, justice, peace, salvation. Finally, a profession is self-governing since anyone who had mastered its art would, by that fact, qualify as one of its members. Knowledge generates an authority not available to the untutored.

Ideals will conflict, so a choice between them becomes unavoidable. Of course, actual performance seldom reaches the ideal. A duty to treat may be compromised by status, power, and money. So-called "late-term abortion" placed the religious ideal above the clinical one. Participation in torture placed national ideal above the clinical one. Scarcity has denied access, keeping caregiver and cared-for apart for lack of status, wealth, or resource.

Catastrophic events further jeopardize a duty to care. For example, a survey of the ethical issues facing the staff at a large university hospital in the event of a flu pandemic showed that nearly one-third found it "professionally acceptable" to "abandon their *workplace* . . . in order to protect themselves and their families." A bare majority, 52 percent, disagreed.[15]

After the SARS outbreak in Canada,

> many of those who treated SARS patients raised concerns about the protections that were provided to safeguard their own health and that of their family members. Conflicting obligations were another significant concern. HCPs [health care professionals] are bound by an ethic of care, therefore, obligations to the patient's well-being should be primary. At the same time, however, HCPs have competing obligations to their families and friends, whom they feared infecting, in addition to obligations to themselves and to their own health (particularly those with special vulnerabilities, such as a co-morbid condition). During SARS, some HCPs questioned their choice of career; indeed, some decided to leave their profession and pursue new ventures, indicating an unwillingness or inability to care for patients in the face of risk. Recent survey data from the U.S. indicate that there exists mixed views on the duty to care for patients during infectious disease outbreaks.[16]

Denying Kant's ethic of duty and the rigor of a classical view of duty, Daniel Sokol writes,

> By virtue of their profession, doctors and nurses have more stringent obligations of beneficence than most. . . . The term "duty of care" refers to these special obligations . . . Its definitional vagueness, combined with its rhetorical appeal, may be used to justify actions without the need for rational deliberation . . . the term may become a subtle instrument of intimidation, pressuring healthcare workers into working in circumstances that they consider morally, psychologically, or physically unacceptable. . . . Are there limits to the duty? Should doctors do everything in their power to benefit their patients? The answer, surely, is no. Doctors are under no moral obligation to donate one of their kidneys to one of their patients, for example. . . . The answer depends, at least in part, on the actual risk to the doctor and the potential benefits (including the alleviation of pain and distress) that his or her presence will bring to the patients.[17]

The modern mood is utilitarian and contractual—some might say realistic. Thus Sokol, and he is not alone, asks for a calculation of risks and benefits in order to determine the caregiver's obligations. Duty thus surrenders the "calling" to prudence.

Democratic values like participation and freedom of choice and the pressures of conflicting roles are well illustrated in the SARS experience. The refusal of many caregivers to treat patients in the early days of the AIDS epidemic is another example. Professional decision-making has been diluted—for example, the near absolute interpretation of patient autonomy in making treatment decisions. The number of "strangers at the bedside" increases, including drug company representatives and business managers. A market ideology revisions caregiving as a commodity, a good to be sold, bought, and consumed. The changing environment increases the likelihood and range of pandemic and, in turn, increases the risks to the caregiver.[18] The context for a duty to care, like so much else in our experience, has grown more threatening.

SHIFTING SANDS

A time of terrorism adds yet more in the way of complexities, conflicts, risks, and threats. Duties grow more various and conflicts between them more unmanageable. Roles multiply, and often the same person is expected to play competing roles simultaneously; for example, treating the victim, restoring the community, protecting against the enemy, preserving the state and society and, not least of all, honoring that in us, human dignity perhaps, that makes sense of both trust and duty. Each role comes with urgent demands, many of which may be felt as having equal weight. None comes with a signal about where it fits into a morally defensible scheme of priorities.

When a "time of terrorism" is framed as a "war on terrorism," things only seem clearer. As in any war, that which defeats the enemy and contributes to victory comes first. In practice, survival of the state claims priority, for it is the agent ultimately responsible for personal, communal, and social survival. Killing, harming, and lying are justified. To be sure, moral limits may be set by the laws of war. But, the ultimate parameters are victory and defeat.

War is a moral temptation. William James, writing nearly one hundred years ago, described it.

> The war against war is going to be no holiday excursion or camping party. The military feelings are too deeply grounded to abdicate their place among our ideals. . . . There is something highly paradoxical in the modern man's relation to war. Ask all our millions, north and south, whether they would vote now . . . to have our war for the Union expunged from history and the record of a peaceful transition . . . substituted for that of its marches and battles, and probably

> hardly a handful of eccentrics would say yes. Those ancestors, those efforts, those memories and legends are the most ideal part of what we now own together, a sacred spiritual possession worth more than all the blood poured out. Yet ask those same people whether they would be willing in cold blood to start another civil war now . . . and not one man or woman would vote for the proposition. . . . Only when forced upon one, only when an enemy's injustice leaves us no alternative, is a war now thought permissible.[19]

And like all temptations, it needs to be put to the critical question: are we in fact in a condition where necessity dictates war? Terrorism, we know, can be differently framed. Indeed, on the record—our own and that of much of global society—"war" is an inapt and inept description, indeed a morally confounding description of what needs to be done and of what can be done in the face of terrorism. So in ending I note once more as I did at the beginning the moral trauma of 9/11. With that, both act and perception were distorted, and distortion now attends ethical judgment and moral practice.

Our experience of catastrophe teaches us that the event—Katrina, SARS, even anthrax—is symptomatic of a chronic and not an acute natural and social condition. Terrorism forecasts a chronic condition, too. Hence, I call it a "time of terrorism," an historic moment when the weak have access to destructive powers and the strong are vulnerable precisely because of their reliance on their size and abilities. Like a mammoth attacking an ant, we flail about, missing the tiny elusive target. Exaggerated by our fears and our rhetoric, by 9/11 in short, we are witness to a psychosocial, even spiritual, effect. Of course, terrorist events will happen, even bioterrorist events will happen, just as hurricanes and earthquakes and floods will happen. As with natural catastrophe, we prepare, encounter, respond, and survive . . . perhaps, we may, even in a time of terrorism, hope and learn to move on.

NOTES

1. "Community Engagement: Leadership Tool for Catastrophic Health Events," Monica Schoch-Spana, Crystal Franco, Jennifer B. Nuzzo, and Christiana Usenza on behalf of the Working Group on Community Engagement in Health Emergency Planning, *Biosecurity and Bioterrorism*, Volume 5, Number 1, 2007.
2. "In Crises, People Tend to Live, or Die, Together," Shankar Vedantam, *D.C. Post*, 9/11/06.
3. "From Ancient Greece to Iraq, the Power of Words in Wartime," Robin Tolmach Lakoff, *NYT*, 5/18/04.
4. "The Terror America Wrought," Robert Scheer, *Truthdig*, 8/7/07.
5. "Why Terrorists Aren't Soldiers," Wesley K. Clark and Kal Raustiala, *NYT*, 8/8/07.
6. See, for example, Alasdair MacIntyre, *After Virtue*, University of Notre Dame Press, Notre Dame, Indiana, 1981. The late Richard Rorty developed, as it were, a

postmodern pragmatism that makes a similar point from a different point of view. In an essay, "Richard Rorty," [*Prospect*, April 2003], Simon Blackburn sums it up,

> But Rorty is, of course, firmly against any attempt to find a foundation for his liberalism. He opposes the tradition which descends from Locke or Kant to recent writers such as Jurgen Habermas and John Rawls, which seeks to prove that a democratic and liberal state is the only rational mode of social organization. For such writers, someone who chose to live in an illiberal or undemocratic state would be trampling on his own reason. It is irrational to sell yourself into the mental servitude that a theocratic state demands. But for Rorty, this Enlightenment attitude with its talk of irrationality is useless. The right pragmatist observation is that theocratic states seem not to work very well, by comparison with liberal democracies—it is theocracies who lose refugees to us, and not vice versa. We can cope, and theocracies cannot.

7. *Counterinsurgency*, FM 3-24, June 2006 (Final Draft). The manual was officially adopted in 2006.

8. Lines 222–31.

9. Lines 345–51.

10. Lines 354–68.

11. The ideological move is not unique to terrorists. Other forms of religious faith, and not just radical Islam, can, but need not, make that move. Thus, Kierkegaard identifies the "man of faith" by the risk of faith, i.e., to leap into the abyss without knowing whether salvation awaits. And the disciple utters, "Lord, I believe, help me in my unbelief."

12. "When Doctors Become Terrorists," Simon Wessely, MD, *NEJM*, published at www.nejm.org. July 16, 2007 (10.1056/NEJMp078149), 7/19/07.

13. *Billy Budd*, a novella begun around 1886 by Herman Melville, was completed but not published before his death. It was discovered in manuscript among Melville's papers in 1924 and published that year.

14. Ludwig Edelstein. "The Hippocratic Oath: Text, Translation and Interpretation," *Bulletin of the History of Medicine*, Supplement 1. Baltimore: Johns Hopkins Press, 1943.

15. "Influenza Pandemic and Professional Duty: Family or Patients First? A Survey of Hospital Employees," Boris P. Ehrenstein, Frank Hanses, and Bernd Salzberge, *BMC Public Health*, 6:311, doi:10.1186/1471-2458-6-311, 10/28/06.

16. "On Pandemics and the Duty to Care: Whose Duty? Who Cares?", *BMC (Biomed Central) Medical Ethics*, Carly Ruderman, C. Shawn Tracy, Cecile M. Bensimon, Mark Bernstein, Laura Hawryluck, Randi Zlotnik Shaul, Ross E. G. Upshur, 7:5, April 2006.

17. "Virulent Epidemics and Scope of Healthcare Workers' Duty of Care," Daniel K. Sokol, *Emerging Infectious Diseases* Vol. 12, No. 8, August 2006, pp. 1238–41.

18. "Infectious diseases are now spreading geographically much faster than at any time in history. It is estimated that 2.1 billion airline passengers traveled in 2006; an outbreak or epidemic in any one part of the world is only a few hours away from becoming an imminent threat somewhere else. Infectious diseases are not only spreading faster, they appear to be emerging more quickly than ever before. Since the 1970s, newly emerging diseases have been identified at the unprecedented rate of one or more per year. There are now nearly forty diseases that were unknown

a generation ago. In addition, during the last five years, WHO has verified more than 1100 epidemic events worldwide." Introduction, World Health Organization Report, *World Health, 2007*, 8/07.

19. "The Moral Equivalent of War," William James, *Essays on Faith and Morals*, World Publishing Company, New York, 1962, pp. 311–12.

Selected Bibliography

Beauchamp, Tom L. and Childress, James F. *Principles of Biomedical Ethics*, Fourth Edition. New York: Oxford University Press, 1994.

Brinkley, Douglas. *The Great Deluge*. New York: HarperCollins, 2006.

Counterinsurgency. Department of Defense, FM 3-24, 2006.

Davis, Mike. *The Monster at Our Door*. New York: The New Press, 2005.

Farmer, Paul. *Pathologies of Power*. Berkeley: University of California Press, 2005.

Friend, David. *Watching the World Change*. New York: Farrar, Straus & Giroux, 2006.

Glassner, Barry. *The Culture of Fear*. Jackson, TN: Basic Books, 1999.

Gostin, Lawrence O. (Editor). *Public Health Law and Ethics*. Berkeley: University of California Press, 2005.

Hoffman, Richard E., Lopez, Wilfredo, Matthews, Gene, Foster, Karen L., Goodman, Richard A. (Editor), Rothstein, Mark A. (Editor). *Law in Public Health Practice*. New York: Oxford University Press, 2003.

Johnson, Steven. *The Ghost Map*. New York: Penguin, 2006.

Leitenberg, Milton. *Assessing the Biological Weapons and Bioterrorism Threat*. Carlisle, PA: Strategic Studies Institute, U.S. Army War College, 2005.

Moreno, Jonathan D. (Editor). *In the Wake of Terror*. Cambridge, MA: MIT Press, 2003.

Mueller, John. *Overblown*. Washington, DC: Free Press, 2006.

Radest, Howard B., Kayman, Harvey, and Richter, Jane. *Ethics and Public Health in an Age of Terrorism*. Columbia: University of South Carolina Center for Public Health Preparedness, 2006.

Radest, Howard B. *Can We Teach Ethics?* Westport, CT: Praeger, 1989.

———. *From Clinic to Classroom: Medical Ethics and Moral Education*. Westport, CT: Praeger, 2000.

Richardson, Louise. *What Terrorists Want*. New York: Random House, 2006.

Rosenberg, Charles E. *The Cholera Years*. Chicago, IL: University of Chicago Press, (1962)1987.

The Small Pox Vaccination Program: Public Health in an Age of Terrorism. Institute of Medicine. Washington, DC: The National Academies Press, 2005.

Ullman, Harlan K. and Wade, James P. *Project Gutenberg's Shock and Awe*. Washington, DC: National Defense University Press, 1996.

Wilson, Richard Ashby (Editor). *Human Rights in the "War on Terror."* New York: Cambridge University Press, 2005.

Wright, Lawrence. *The Looming Tower*. New York: Alfred A. Knopf, 2006.

JOURNALS

AJOB—American Journal of Bioethics
Annals of Emergency Medicine
Biosecurity Briefing, University of Pittsburgh
BMC—BioMed Central
BMJ—Journal of the British Medical Association
CMAJ—Journal of the Canadian Medical Association
Emerging Infectious Diseases
Emerging Themes in Epidemiology
Hastings Center Report
Health Affairs
JAMA—Journal of the American Medical Association
Journal of Homeland Security, Department of Homeland Security
Kennedy Institute of Ethics Journal
The Lancet
NEJM, New England Journal of Medicine
NYT—New York Times
SSI—Strategic Studies Institute, U.S. Army War College
Washington Post

OTHER REFERENCES

Agencies and Organizations

American Public Health Association
CDC—Center for Disease Control
Center for Law and the Public's Health, Georgetown and Johns Hopkins
CIA—Central Intelligence Agency
Department of Homeland Security
Federation of American Scientists

FEMA—Federal Emergency Management Agency
Find Law
HHS—Department of Health and Human Services
National Counterterrorism Center
PLOS—Public Library of Science
UNESCO—The United Nations Educational, Scientific and Cultural Organization
WHO—World Health Organization

Film

When the Levees Broke: A Requiem in Four Acts. Spike Lee, 40 Acres & a Mule Filmworks Production. (Teaching the Levees, Teachers College, Columbia University, The Rockefeller Foundation, HBO Documentary Films, Teachers College Press, and the EdLab)

Index

About the Author

Howard B. Radest is the dean emeritus of The Humanist Institute, a member of the National Council of Ethical Culture Leaders, and a former member of the Board of the Association for Moral Education. He is a member of the Highlands Institute for American Religious and Philosophic Thought. He serves on the Advisory Committee of the Appignani Center for Bioethics. He is a senior fellow of the Center for Inquiry.

From 1979–1991 he served as director [headmaster] of The Ethical Culture Fieldston School in New York City. Prior to that he was professor of philosophy and director of the School of American Studies at Ramapo College in New Jersey (1970–1979). He was adjunct professor of philosophy at Fairleigh Dickenson University, at The Union Graduate School and most recently at The University of South Carolina-Beaufort where he taught medical ethics, comparative religion, and social and political philosophy. He served as ethics consultant to Hilton Head Hospital and chair of its Biomedical Ethics Committee. He is an emeritus consulting member of the SC Medical Assn Ethics Committee. He is consultant to the Center for Preparedness, School of Public Health, University of South Carolina. He was executive director of The American Ethical Union (1963–1969) and leader of the Ethical Culture Society of Bergen County, New Jersey (1956–1963).

Dr. Radest was the founder and first chair (1983–1991) of the University Seminar on Moral Education, Columbia University. He is a member of the Board of the North American Committee for Humanism (NACH). He served from 1978–1988 as co-chair of The International Humanist and Ethical Union. He is on the editorial boards of *The Humanist* and *Religious Humanism*.

In addition to his numerous articles, his books are *Toward Common Ground* (Ungar, 1968), a history of the Ethical Culture Movement in the United States, *Can We Teach Ethics?* (Praeger, 1989), *The Devil and Secular Humanism* (Praeger, 1990), *Community Service, Encounter With Strangers* (Praeger, 1993), *Humanism With A Human Face* (Praeger, 1996), *Felix Adler: An Ethical Culture,* (Peter Lang, Publishers, 1998), *From Clinic To Classroom—Medical Ethics and Moral Education,* (Praeger, 2000), *Biomedical Ethics,* editor, (Prometheus, 2007), *Ethics and Public Health in a Time of Terror* [The Center for Preparedness [CDC] at the School of Public Health, University of South Carolina], *Bioethics: Catastrophes in a Time of Terror* [Lexington, 2009].

Dr. Radest received his B.A. at Columbia College, his M.A. in philosophy and psychology at The New School for Social Research and his Ph.D. in philosophy at Columbia University. He is a member of the American Society for Bioethics and Humanities, the Society for the Advancement of American Philosophy, and of Phi Beta Kappa. He received the Distinguished Service Award (1994) of The Humanist Institute, The Distinguished Service Award (1993) of the American Humanist Association, The Kuhmerker Award (1988) of The Moral Education Association, and was a Cornell Scholar and a Hillman Scholar. He is listed in *Who's Who* and *Who's Who in Education.*

www.ingramcontent.com/pod-product-compliance
Lightning Source LLC
Chambersburg PA
CBHW051252200926
51612CB00001B/13
* 9 7 8 0 7 3 9 1 3 5 2 7 3 *